Surgery: Complications, Risks and Consequences

Series Editor
Brendon J. Coventry

For further volumes:
http://www.springer.com/series/11761

Brendon J. Coventry

Editor

Cardio-Thoracic, Vascular, Renal and Transplant Surgery

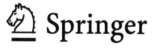 Springer

Editor
Brendon J. Coventry, BMBS, PhD,
FRACS, FACS, FRSM
Discipline of Surgery
Royal Adelaide Hospital
University of Adelaide
Adelaide, SA
Australia

ISBN 978-1-4471-7085-3   ISBN 978-1-4471-5418-1   (eBook)
DOI 10.1007/978-1-4471-5418-1
Springer London Heidelberg New York Dordrecht

Printed on acid-free paper

Springer is part of Springer Science+Business Media (www.springer.com)

This book is dedicated to my wonderful wife Christine and children Charles, Cameron, Alexander and Eloise who make me so proud, having supported me through this mammoth project; my patients, past, present and future; my numerous mentors, teachers, colleagues, friends and students, who know who they are; my parents Beryl and Lawrence; and my parents-in-law Barbara and George, all of whom have taught me and encouraged me to achieve

"Without love and understanding we have but nothing"

Brendon J. Coventry

Foreword I

This comprehensive treatise is remarkable for its breadth and scope and its authorship by global experts. Indeed, knowledge of its content is essential if we are to achieve optimal and safe outcomes for our patients. The content embodies the details of our surgical discipline and how to incorporate facts and evidence into our surgical judgment as well as recommendations to our patients.

While acknowledging that the technical aspects of surgery are its distinguishing framework of our profession, the art and judgment of surgery requires an in depth knowledge of biology, anatomy, pathophysiology, clinical science, surgical outcomes and complications that distinguishes the theme of this book. This knowledge is essential to assure us that we are we doing the right operation, at the right time, and in the right patient. In turn, that knowledge is essential to take into account how surgical treatment interfaces with the correct sequence and combination with other treatment modalities. It is also essential to assess the extent of scientific evidence from clinical trials and surgical expertise that is the underpinning of our final treatment recommendation to our patient.

Each time I sit across from a patient to make a recommendation for a surgical treatment, I am basing my recommendation on a "benefit/risk ratio" that integrates scientific evidence, and my intuition gained through experience. That is, do the potential benefits outweigh the potential risks and complications as applied to an individual patient setting? The elements of that benefit/ risk ratio that are taken into account include: the natural history of the disease, the stage/extent of disease, scientific and empirical evidence of treatment outcomes, quality of life issues (as perceived by the patient), co-morbidity that might influence surgical outcome, risks and complications inherent to the operation (errors of commission) and the risk(s) of not proceeding with an operation (errors of omission).

Thus, if we truly want to improve our surgical outcomes, then we must understand and be able to either avoid, or execute sound management of, any complications that occur (regardless of whether they are due to co-morbidity or iatrogenic causes), to get our patent safely through the operation and its post-operative course. These subjects are nicely incorporated into the content of this book.

I highly recommend this book as a practical yet comprehensive treatise for the practicing surgeon and the surgical trainee. It is well organized, written with great clarity and nicely referenced when circumstances require further information.

Charles M. Balch, MD, FACS
Professor of Surgery
University of Texas, Southwestern Medical Center,
Dallas, TX, USA
Formerly, Professor of Surgery, Johns Hopkins Hospital,
Baltimore, MD, USA
Formerly, Executive Vice President and CEO,
American Society of Clinical Oncology (ASCO)
Past-President, Society of Surgical Oncology (USA)

Foreword II

Throughout my clinical academic career I have aspired to improve the quality and safety of my surgical and clinical practice. It is very clear, while reading this impressive collection and synthesis of high-impact clinical evidence and international expert consensus, that in this new textbook, Brendon Coventry has the ambition to innovate and advance the quality and safety of surgical discipline.

In these modern times, where we find an abundance of information that is available through the internet, and of often doubtful authenticity, it is vital that we retain a professional responsibility for the collection, analysis and dissemination of evidenced-based and accurate knowledge and guidance to benefit both clinicians and our patients.

This practical and broad-scoped compendium, which contains over 250 procedures and their related complications and associated risks, will undoubtedly become a benchmark to raise the safety and quality of surgical practice for all that read it. It also manages to succeed in providing a portal for all surgeons, at any stage of their careers, to reflect on the authors' own combined experiences and the collective insights of a strong and influential network of peers.

This text emphasizes the need to understand and appreciate our patients and the intimate relationship that their physiology, co-morbidities and underlying diagnosis can have upon their unique surgical risk with special regard to complications and adverse events.

I recognize that universally across clinical practice and our profession, the evidence base and guidance to justify our decision-making is growing, but there is also a widening gap between what we know and what we do. The variation that we see in the quality of practice throughout the world should not be tolerated.

This text makes an assertive contribution to promote quality by outlining the prerequisite foundational knowledge of surgery, science and anatomy and their complex interactions with clinical outcome that is needed for all in the field of surgery.

I thoroughly recommend this expertly constructed collection. Its breadth and quality is a testament to its authors and editor.

Lord Ara Darzi, PC, KBE, FRCS, FRS
Paul Hamlyn Chair of Surgery
Imperial College London, London, UK
Formerly Undersecretary of State for Health,
Her Majesty's Government, UK

Conditions of Use and Disclaimer

Information is provided *for improved medical education and potential improvement in clinical practice only*. The information is based on composite material from research studies and professional personal opinion and does not guarantee accuracy for any specific clinical situation or procedure. There is also *no express or implied guarantee to accuracy or that surgical complications will be prevented, minimized, or reduced* in any way. The advice is *intended for use by individuals with suitable professional qualifications* and education in medical practice and the ability to apply the knowledge in a suitable manner for a specific condition or disease, and in an appropriate clinical context. The data is complex by nature and open to some interpretation. The purpose is to assist medical practitioners to improve awareness of possible complications, risks or consequences associated with surgical procedures for the benefit of those practitioners in the improved care of their patients. The application of the information contained herein for a specific patient or problem must be performed with care to ensure that the situation and advice is appropriate and correct for that patient and situation. The material is expressly *not for medico-legal purposes*.

The information contained in *Surgery: Complications, Risks and Consequences* is provided for the purpose of improving consent processes in healthcare and in no way guarantees prevention, early detection, risk reduction, economic benefit or improved practice of surgical treatment of any disease or condition.

The information provided in *Surgery: Complications, Risks and Consequences* is of a general nature and is not a substitute for independent medical advice or research in the management of particular diseases or patient situations by health care professionals. It should not be taken as replacing or overriding medical advice.

The Publisher or *Copyright* holder does not accept any liability for any injury, loss, delay or damage incurred arising from use, misuse, interpretation, omissions or reliance on the information provided in *Surgery: Complications, Risks and Consequences* directly or indirectly.

Currency and Accuracy of Information

The user should always check that any information acted upon is up-to-date and accurate. Information is provided in good faith and is **subject to change and alteration without notice**. Every effort is made with *Surgery: Complications, Risks and Consequences* to provide current information, but no warranty, guarantee or legal responsibility is given that information provided or referred to has not changed without the knowledge of the publisher, editor or authors. Always check the quality of information provided or referred to for accuracy for the situation where it is intended to be used, or applied. We do, however, attempt to provide useful and valid information. Because of the broad nature of the information provided incompleteness or omissions of specific or general complications may have occured and users must take this into account when using the text. No responsibility is taken for delayed, missed or inaccurate diagnosis of any illness, disease or health state at any time.

External Web Site Links or References

The decisions about the accuracy, currency, reliability and correctness of information made by individuals using the *Surgery: Complications, Risks and Consequences* information or from external Internet links remain the individuals own concern and responsibility. Such external links or reference materials or other information should not be taken as an endorsement, agreement or recommendation of any third party products, services, material, information, views or content offered by these sites or publications. Users should check the sources and validity of information obtained for themselves prior to use.

Privacy and Confidentiality

We maintain confidentiality and privacy of personal information but do not guarantee any confidentiality or privacy.

Errors or Suggested Changes

If you or any colleagues note any errors or wish to suggest changes please notify us directly as they would be gratefully received.

How to Use This Book

This book provides a resource for better understanding of surgical procedures and potential complications in general terms. The application of this material will depend on the individual patient and clinical context. It is not intended to be absolutely comprehensive for all situations or for all patients, but act as a 'guide' for understanding and prediction of complications, to assist in risk management and improvement of patient outcomes.

The design of the book is aimed at:

- Reducing Risk and better Managing Risks associated with surgery
- Providing information about 'general complications' associated with surgery
- Providing information about 'specific complications' associated with surgery
- Providing comprehensive information in one location, to assist surgeons in their explanation to the patient during the consent process

For each specific surgical procedure the text provides:

- Description and some background of the surgical procedure
- Anatomical points and possible variations
- Estimated Frequencies
- Perspective
- Major Complications

From this, a better understanding of the risks, complications and consequences associated with surgical procedures can hopefully be gained by the clinician for explanation of relevant and appropriate aspects to the patient.

The *Estimated frequency lists are not mean't to be totally comprehensive* or to contain all of the information that needs to be explained in obtaining informed consent from the patient for a surgical procedure. Indeed, *most of the information is for the surgeon* or reader only, *not designed for the patient*, however, parts should be selected by the surgeon at their discretion for appropriate explanation to the individual patient in the consent process.

Many patients would not understand or would be confused by the number of potential complications that may be associated with a specific surgical procedure, so ___some degree of selective discussion of the risks, complications and consequences would be necessary and advisable,___ as would usually occur in clinical practice. This judgement should necessarily be left to the surgeon, surgeon-in-training or other practitioner.

Preface

Over the last decade or so we have witnessed a rapid change in the consumer demand for information by patients preparing for a surgical procedure. This is fuelled by multiple factors including the 'internet revolution', altered public consumer attitudes, professional patient advocacy, freedom of information laws, insurance issues, risk management, and medicolegal claims made through the legal system throughout the western world, so that the need has arisen for a higher, fairer and clearer standard of *'informed consent'*.

One of the my main difficulties encountered as a young intern, and later as a surgical resident, registrar and consultant surgeon, was obtaining information for use for the pre-operative consenting of patients, and for managing patients on the ward after surgical operations. I watched others struggle with the same problem too. The literature contained many useful facts and clinical studies, but it was unwieldy and very time-consuming to access, and the information that was obtained seemed specific to well-defined studies of highly specific groups of patients. These patient studies, while useful, often did not address my particular patient under treatment in the clinic, operating theatre or ward. Often the studies came from centres with vast experience of a particular condition treated with one type of surgical procedure, constituting a series or trial.

What I wanted to know was:

- The **main complications** associated with a surgical procedure;
- **Information that could be provided** during the consent process, and
- How to **reduce the relative risks** of a complication, where possible

This information was difficult to find in one place!

As a young surgeon, on a very long flight from Adelaide to London, with much time to think and fuelled by some very pleasant champagne, I started making some notes about how I might tackle this problem. My first draft was idle scribble, as I listed the ways surgical complications could be classified. After finding over 10 different classification systems for listing complications, the task became much larger and more complex. I then realized why someone had not taken on this job before!

After a brief in-flight sleep and another glass, the task became far less daunting and suddenly much clearer – the champagne was very good, and there was little else to do in any case!

It was then that I decided to speak with as many of my respected colleagues as I could from around the globe, to get their opinions and advice. The perspectives that emerged were remarkable, as many of them had faced the same dilemmas in their own practices and hospitals, also without a satisfactory solution.

What developed was a composite documentation of information (i) from the published literature and (ii) from the opinions of many experienced surgical practitioners in the field – to provide a text to supply information on **Complications, Risks and Consequences of Surgery** for surgical and other clinical practitioners to use at the bedside and in the clinic.

This work represents the culmination of more than 10 years work with the support and help of colleagues from around the world, for the benefit of their students, junior surgical colleagues, peers, and patients. To them, I owe much gratitude for their cooperation, advice, intellect, experience, wise counsel, friendship and help, for their time, and for their continued encouragement in this rather long-term and complex project. I have already used the text material myself with good effect and it has helped me enormously in my surgical practice.

The text aims to provide health professionals with useful information, which can be selectively used to better inform patients of the potential surgical complications, risks and consequences. I sincerely hope it fulfils this role.

Adelaide, SA, Australia   Brendon J. Coventry, BMBS, PhD,
                                                          FRACS, FACS, FRSM

Acknowledgments

I wish to thank:

The many learned friends and experienced colleagues who have contributed in innumerable ways along the way in the writing of this text.

Professor Sir Peter Morris, formerly Professor of Surgery at Oxford University, and also Past-President of the College of Surgeons of England, for allowing me to base my initial work at the Nuffield Department of Surgery (NDS) and John Radcliffe Hospital in the University of Oxford, for the UK sector of the studies. He and his colleagues have provided encouragement and valuable discussion time over the course of the project.

The (late) Professor John Farndon, Professor of Surgery at the University of Bristol, Bristol Royal Infirmary, UK; and Professor Robert Mansel, Professor of Surgery at the University of Wales, Cardiff, UK for discussions and valued advice.

Professor Charles Balch, then Professor of Surgery at the Johns Hopkins University, Baltimore, Maryland, USA, and Professor Clifford Ko, from UCLA and American College of Surgeons NSQIP Program, USA, for helpful discussions.

Professor Armando Guiliano, formerly of the John Wayne Cancer Institute, Santa Monica, California, USA for his contributions and valuable discussions.

Professor Jonathan Meakins, then Professor of Surgery at McGill University, Quebec, Canada, who provided helpful discussions and encouragement, during our respective sabbatical periods, which coincided in Oxford; and later as Professor of Surgery at Oxford University.

Over the last decade, numerous clinicians have discussed and generously contributed their experience to the validation of the range and relative frequency of complications associated with the wide spectrum of surgical procedures. These clinicians include:

Los Angeles, USA: Professor Carmack Holmes, Cardiothoracic Surgeon, Los Angeles (UCLA); Professor Donald Morton, Melanoma Surgeon, Los Angeles; Dr R Essner, Melanoma Surgeon, Los Angeles.

New York, USA: Professor Murray Brennan; Dr David Jacques; Prof L Blumgart; Dr Dan Coit; Dr Mary Sue Brady (Surgeons, Department of Surgery, Memorial Sloan-Kettering Cancer Centre, New York);

Oxford, UK: Dr Linda Hands, Vascular Surgeon; Dr Jack Collin, Vascular Surgeon; Professor Peter Friend, Transplant and Vascular Surgeon; Dr Nick Maynard, Upper Gastrointestinal Surgeon; Dr Mike Greenall, Breast Surgeon; Dr Jane Clark, Breast Surgeon; Professor Derek Gray, Vascular/Pancreatic Surgeon; Dr Julian Britton, Hepato-Biliary Surgeon; Dr Greg Sadler, Endocrine Surgeon; Dr Christopher Cunningham, Colorectal Surgeon; Professor Neil Mortensen, Colorectal Surgeon; Dr Bruce George, Colorectal Surgeon; Dr Chris Glynn, Anaesthetist. (National Health Service (NHS), Oxford, UK).

Bristol, UK: Professor Derek Alderson.

Adelaide, Australia: Professor Guy Ludbrook, Anesthetist; Dr Elizabeth Tam, Anesthetist.

A number of senior medical students at the University of Adelaide, including Hwee Sim Tan, Adelaine S Lam, Ramon Pathi, Mohd Azizan Ghzali, William Cheng, Sue Min Ooi, Teena Silakong, and Balaji Rajacopalin, who assisted during their student projects in the preliminary feasibility studies and research, and their participation is much appreciated. Thanks also to numerous sixth year students, residents and surgeons at Hospitals in Adelaide who participated in questionnaires and surveys.

The support of the University of Adelaide, especially the Department of Surgery, and Royal Adelaide Hospital has been invaluable in allowing the sabbatical time to engineer the collaborations necessary for this project to progress. I thank Professors Glyn Jamieson and Guy Maddern for their support in this regard.

I especially thank the Royal Australasian College of Surgeons for part support through the Marjorie Hooper Fellowship.

I thank my clinical colleagues on the Breast, Endocrine and Surgical Oncology Unit at the Royal Adelaide Hospital, especially Grantley Gill, James Kollias and Melissa Bochner, for caring for my patients and assuming greater clinical load when I have been away.

Professor Bill Runciman, Australian Patient Safety Foundation, for all of his advice and support; Professors Cliff Hughes and Bruce Barraclough, from the Royal Australasian College of Surgeons, the Clinical Excellence Commission, New South Wales, and the Australian Commission (Council) on Safety and Quality in Healthcare.

Thanks too to Kai Holt and Carrie Cooper who helped to organise me and my work. I also acknowledge my collaborator Martin Ashdown for being so patient during distractions from our scientific research work. Also to Graeme Cogdell, Imagart Design Ltd, Adelaide, for his expertise and helpful discussions.

Importantly, I truly appreciate and thank my wife Christine, my four children and our parents/ wider family for their support in every way towards seeing this project through to its completion, and in believing so much in me, and in my work.

Adelaide, SA, Australia   Brendon J. Coventry, BMBS, PhD,
                                                                        FRACS, FACS, FRSM

Contents

Contributors

Jayme Bennetts Cardiac and Thoracic Surgery, Flinders Medical Centre, Adelaide, Australia

John Chen South Australian Liver Transplant Unit, Flinders Medical Centre, Adelaide, Australia

Brendon J. Coventry Discipline of Surgery, Royal Adelaide Hospital, University of Adelaide, Adelaide, SA, Australia

James Edwards Department of Surgery, Royal Adelaide Hospital, Adelaide, Australia

Jonathon Fawcett Queensland Liver Transplant Service, Princess Alexandra Hospital, Brisbane, Australia

Robert Fitridge Discipline of Surgery, The Queen Elizabeth Hospital, Woodville, Australia

Oliver Hakenberg Department of Urology, University Hospital, Rostock University, Rostock, Germany

Craig Jurisevic Department of Surgery, Royal Adelaide Hospital, Adelaide, Australia

David King Department of Vascular Surgery, Royal Adelaide Hospital, Adelaide, Australia

Villis Marshall Discipline of Surgery, The University of Adelaide, Royal Adelaide Hospital, Adelaide, Australia

John Miller Department of Surgery, Queen Elizabeth Hospital, Adelaide, Australia

Peter Morris University of Oxford, Oxford, UK

Christine Russell Central and Northern Adelaide Renal and Transplantation Service, Royal Adelaide Hospital, Adelaide, Australia

John Walsh Discipline of Surgery, The Flinders University of South Australia, Adelaide, Australia

Chapter 1
Introduction

Brendon J. Coventry

This volume deals with complications, risks, and consequences related to a range of procedures under the broad headings of vascular surgery, including sympathectomy, amputation and vascular access surgery, thoracic surgery, cardiac surgery, renal surgery, and renal and liver transplant surgery.

Important Note

It should be emphasized that the risks and frequencies that are given here *represent derived figures*. These *figures are best estimates of relative frequencies across most institutions*, not merely the highest-performing ones, and as such are often representative of a number of studies, which include different patients with differing comorbidities and different surgeons. In addition, the risks of complications in lower or higher risk patients may lie outside these estimated ranges, and individual clinical judgement is required as to the expected risks communicated to the patient, staff, or for other purposes. The range of risks is also derived from experience and the literature; while risks outside this range may exist, certain risks may be reduced or absent due to variations of procedures or surgical approaches. It is recognized that different patients, practitioners, institutions, regions and countries may vary in their requirements and recommendations.

Individual clinical judgement should always be exercised, of course, when applying the general information contained in these documents to individual patients in a clinical setting.

B.J. Coventry, BMBS, PhD, FRACS, FACS, FRSM
Discipline of Surgery, Royal Adelaide Hospital, University of Adelaide,
L5 Eleanor Harrald Building, North Terrace, 5000 Adelaide, SA, Australia
e-mail: brendon.coventry@adelaide.edu.au

B.J. Coventry (ed.), *Cardio-Thoracic, Vascular, Renal and Transplant Surgery*,
Surgery: Complications, Risks and Consequences,
DOI 10.1007/978-1-4471-5418-1_1, © Springer-Verlag London 2014

The authors would like to thank the following experienced clinicians who discussed the chapters and acted as advisors: Professor Jack Collin, Oxford, United Kingdom, and Dr. Linda Hands, Oxford, United Kingdom; Dr. E Carmack Holmes, Snr, Head of Cardiac Surgery & Surgery, UCLA, Los Angeles, USA; and Professor Peter Friend, Oxford, UK.

Chapter 2
Blood Transfusion

Brendon J. Coventry

General Perspective and Overview

Blood transfusion and the use of blood product has been carefully reassessed from the pre-HIV period when blood was more readily transfused for a variety of conditions and at threshold levels that were vastly different from the practices of today. Some of this impetus for change has come from the risk of blood-borne diseases such as HIV, prion slow-virus diseases, and hepatitis, while another important aspect has arisen from the sheer demands and costs of transfusion services, together with the necessity to separate blood products into the many components that can be more selectively and wisely used. Yet another facet is the increasing awareness that transfusion either too early or too rapidly can *cause* a range of serious and economically costly complications, which can worsen the prognosis and outcomes of patients. Transfusion was often indicated in the past for otherwise well patients with hemoglobin (Hb) levels less than 100 g/l (10 g/dL). The current practice in many institutions throughout the world is for transfusion to be considered when the hemoglobin falls below 70 g/l or when the patient becomes symptomatic (even at higher Hb levels).

The commonest problems causing complications for blood transfusions remain those of human error, especially concerning labeling of the patient, the patient blood sample, the intra-laboratory standards, and the correct administration of the correct blood to the correct patient.

With these factors and facts in mind, the information given in these chapters must be appropriately and discernibly interpreted and used.

The **use of specialized blood collection, labeling, crossmatching, and processing units with standardized care** is essential to the success of the blood

B.J. Coventry, BMBS, PhD, FRACS, FACS, FRSM
Discipline of Surgery, Royal Adelaide Hospital, University of Adelaide,
L5 Eleanor Harrald Building, North Terrace, 5000 Adelaide, SA, Australia
e-mail: brendon.coventry@adelaide.edu.au

B.J. Coventry (ed.), *Cardio-Thoracic, Vascular, Renal and Transplant Surgery*,
Surgery: Complications, Risks and Consequences,
DOI 10.1007/978-1-4471-5418-1_2, © Springer-Verlag London 2014

transfusion process overall and can significantly reduce risk of complications or aid early detection, prompt intervention, and cost.

Important Note

It should be emphasized that the risks and frequencies that are given here *represent derived figures*. These *figures are best estimates of relative frequencies across most institutions*, not merely the highest-performing ones, and as such are often representative of a number of studies, which include different patients with differing comorbidities and different surgeons. In addition, the risks of complications in lower- or higher-risk patients may lie outside these estimated ranges, and individual clinical judgement is required as to the expected risks communicated to the patient, staff, or for other purposes. The range of risks is also derived from experience and the literature; while risks outside this range may exist, certain risks may be reduced or absent due to variations of procedures or surgical approaches. It is recognized that different patients, practitioners, institutions, regions and countries may vary in their requirements and recommendations.

Allogeneic Blood and Blood Product Transfusion

Description

Usually no anesthesia is required, but local anesthetic may be used on occasions. The aim is to transfuse compatible blood, or blood components, via a vein into the patient to replenish the amount of blood or blood components in a patient. Careful identification of the blood type, date of expiry, and patient is very important to ensure the correctly compatible blood is being transfused to the correct patient. Human error remains the most common complication with transfusion of blood or blood components. The relative risk(s) of transfusion of blood or blood products always needs to be carefully evaluated against the risk(s) of not transfusing the patient. Red cell transfusion is rarely necessary until the hemoglobin is <70 g/l, unless the patient is symptomatic or other indications exist. Age is a relative indication, although the risk of cardiac failure and any sequelae of transfusion reactions, should they occur, should be considered against the relative risk to the elderly patient of a low hemoglobin level, dependent on the cause. A useful discussion and further advice is provided in the NHMRC Guidelines on the use of blood products referenced below.

Anatomical Points

Venous access is usually by an arm vein, often the cephalic or brachial vein within the cubital fossa. The anatomy of the venous system is highly variable throughout

Table 2.1 Complications of blood transfusion and blood product transfusion

Complications, risks, and consequences	Estimated frequency
Most significant/serious complications	
Fever (mild, moderate, high)[a]	5–20 %
Myocardial problems (cardiac failure, infarction)[a]	1–5 %
Renal failure[a]	1–5 %
Jaundice[a]	1–5 %
Immunological cross priming[a] (immunization; cellular activation or tolerance induction)	1–5 %
Rare significant/serious problems	
Infection (bacterial, fungal, viral, other)	
Cellulitis	0.1–1 %
Systemic	<0.1 %
Disseminated intravascular coagulation[a]	<0.1 %
Incompatibility with other fluids[a]	0.1–1 %
Intravascular hemolysis[a]	0.1–1 %
White blood cell incompatibility[a]	0.1–1 %
Air embolism[a]	<0.1 %
Multisystem organ failure[a]	0.1–1 %
Death[a]	<0.1 %
Less serious complications	
Extravasation	0.1–1 %
Skin rash	5–20 %

[a]Dependent on the situation, underlying pathology, anatomy, comorbidities, surgical technique, and preferences

the body, and those in the arm are no exception. The most constant vein is the cephalic vein, which is sometimes used for a venous cut-down procedure at the radial aspect of the wrist, the lateral aspect of the cubital fossa, or in the delto-pectoral groove. The basilic vein is often used for infusion of blood, and occasion-ally a transverse cubital fossa vein is often present and used. These may be visible, but are often more easily palpated. Central venous access is sometimes required or preferable, especially in very unwell patients, often in the intensive care unit setting or when peripheral veins are difficult to cannulate. Occasionally, infusion port insertion is useful for CV line administration of repeated transfusions of blood or blood components.

Perspective

See Tables 2.1 and 2.2. Transfusion of blood is a relatively safe procedure in most cases, provided that the correct collection, crossmatching, labeling, and patient identification protocols are followed. However, minor problems are not uncom-mon, especially when multiple or very rapid, large transfusions are used. White cell transfusions are associated with higher incidence of transfusion reactions, in general. Transfusion reactions include a spectrum ranging from low-grade fever, rash, and severe urticaria to intravascular coagulation, cardiovascular collapse,

Table 2.2 Noninfectious risks and complications of transfusion

Risk	Estimated frequency
Earlier complications: immediate to hours	
Fever nonhemolytic, non-septic transfusion reaction	0.1–1 %
Volume circulatory overload[a]	1–5 %
Hemolysis	<0.1 %
Transfusion acute pulmonary injury	< 0.1 %
Allergic reaction – mild, moderate	1–5 %
Allergic reaction – severe anaphylaxis	<0.1 %
Extravasation of transfusate[a]	0.1–1 %
Electrolyte problems[a]	Individual
Coagulation problems[a]	Individual
Later complications: days to months	
Antibodies to RBC	
1–6 RBC transfusions[c]	0.1–1 %
>6 RBC transfusions[c] (causing delayed and difficult crossmatching; rarely delayedintravascular hemolysis)	5–20 %
Iron overload (chronic repetitive RBC transfusions only)[b]	>80 %
Immunosuppression[d] (may contribute to mortality, infection, malignant recurrence or progression, better graft tolerance)	50–80 %
Anti-HLA antibodies[d] (thrombocytopenia, tissue matching difficulties)	5–20 %
Antiplatelet antibodies[d] (thrombocytopenia, purpura)	1–5 %
Graft-vs.-host disease[d]	<0.1 %
Venous access problems (with repetitive transfusions)[c]	50–80 %

Adapted from Eder .and Chambers (2007), with permission

Note: (i) The incidence of many of the above transfusion reactions of each type is often associated with the blood component transfused (packed washed RBC, whole blood, platelets, clotting factors, plasma), the purity of separation and the quality of pre-transfusion screening, and (ii) the assumption of high level and high quality crossmatching, compatibility testing, and patient identification procedures prior to transfusion

RBC red blood cells

[a]Increased with and related to age and comorbidities of the transfused patient

[b]Dependent on the situation, underlying pathology, anatomy, comorbidities, surgical technique, and preferences

[c]Often related to exposure to minor antigens and immunological responsiveness

[d]Related to underlying disease, comorbidities, and immune status

intravascular hemolysis, jaundice, severe anaphylaxis, and rarely death. Most transfusion reactions are minor in nature and can be treated with simple measures. Stopping the transfusion immediately a transfusion reaction is suspected or proven is usually wise. Blood replacement is typically achieved with the use of washed, packed red blood cells or more rarely whole blood, especially in the rapid hemorrhage setting, for urgent blood replacement, for example, after trauma, or during torrential intraoperative hemorrhage. The transfusion of blood products includes platelets, fresh frozen plasma, and cryopreserved clotting factors. Rarely, while blood cells are transfused, but these carry the highest risk of a transfusion reaction, principally due to the multiple membrane-bound foreign antigens and transfusion of primed dendritic and T cells. Severe reactions are essentially almost avoidable through careful crossmatching, accurate identification, and diligent administration of blood. The use of washed, packed red blood cells has also led to a reduction in the incidence of transfusion reactions. Infection is very rare, and unused blood, especially when un-refridgerated for over 3 h, should be appropriately labeled and returned to the transfusion laboratory to be discarded. Among the most common related problems, especially in the elderly, is fluid overload either through direct volume infusion or osmotic "expansion" of the intravascular compartment due to the drawing in of fluid by the hyperosmolar blood and products. The nature of augmentation or suppression of immune responses by transfusion, which are also potential related problems, is not particularly well understood currently.

Major Complications

Human error remains the main cause for **transfusion incompatibility** and is the most common complication with transfusion of blood. Major **transfusion reactions** include **high fever and rigors, intravascular coagulation, cardiovascular collapse, intravascular hemolysis, jaundice**, and **severe anaphylaxis. Infection** of blood before or during transfusion is very rare. **Drip site skin infection** is more common with prolonged IV cannulation >72 h and immunosuppression, but relatively rare with short-term cannulation. **Air embolism** requires a large amount of air to produce symptoms and is very rare, but catastrophic when it occurs. These are all rare, with careful blood administration. **Death** from transfusion reactions is exceedingly rare, but is reported. More common is circulatory overload producing **cardiac failure**, especially in elderly patients with preexisting comorbidities. In situations where fluid overload may occur, the careful use of concomitant diuretics can reduce risk of cardiac failure. Transfusion-induced immunosuppression and immune augmentation are potential effects. **Incompatibility** of other fluids with blood should be checked for prior to combination of any nonstandard fluid to be administered through the same or a joined IV line.

Consent and Risk Reduction

Main Points to Explain

- Discomfort
- Bleeding
- Transfusion reaction
- Hematological problems
- Infection
- Risks without transfusion

Further Reading, References, and Resources

Benhamou D, Lienhart A, Auroy Y, Péquignot F, Jougla E. Accidents by ABO incompatibility and
    other main complications related to blood transfusion in surgical patients: data from the French
    national survey on anaesthesia-related deaths. Transfus Clin Biol. 2005;12(5):389–90.
de Saint MG, Pequignot F, Auroy Y, Aouba A, Benhamou D, Jougla E, Lienhart A. Patient blood
    management and transfusion. Anesthesiology. 2009;111(2):444–5. author reply 445–6.
Eder AF, Chambers LA. Noninfectious complications of blood transfusion. Arch Pathol Lab Med.
    2007;131:708–18 [Note: This is an excellent reference for more detail].
**NHMRC Clinical Practice Guidelines on the Use of Blood Components (red blood cells,
    platelets, fresh frozen plasma, cryoprecipitate)** © Commonwealth of Australia, 2002 ISBN
    Print: 1864961449 Online: 1864961384
NHMRC web address: http://www.nhmrc.health.gov.au
[Note: These guidelines are excellent reference point and are a joint initiative of the National
    Health and Medical Research Council and the Australasian Society of Blood Transfusion, in
    cooperation with the Commonwealth Department of Health and Ageing, the Royal Australasian
    College of Surgeons, the Australian and New Zealand College of Anaesthetists, and other
    relevant groups.]

Chapter 3
Arterial Surgery

**David King, Robert Fitridge, Christine Russell,
John Walsh, Craig Jurisevic, and Brendon J. Coventry**

Vascular Surgical Procedures: General Perspective and Overview

The relative risks and complications increase proportionately according to the site of vascular disease, dissection, or anastomosis within the vascular system. This is principally related to the surgical accessibility, ability to correct the problem, blood supply, risk of tissue/organ injury, hematoma formation, and technical ease of surgery, including achieving an anastomosis when desired.

The main serious complications are **bleeding and infection,** which can be minimized by the adequate exposure, mobilization, reduction of tension, and ensuring satisfactory blood supply to the distal tissues. Infection is the main sequel of poor tissue perfusion or hematoma formation and may lead to **abscess**

D. King, BmedSc, MBBS, FRACS (GenSrg/Vasc) (✉)
Department of Vascular Surgery, Royal Adelaide Hospital, Adelaide, Australia
e-mail: davidking@internode.on.net

R. Fitridge, MBBS, MS, FRACS
Discipline of Surgery, The Queen Elizabeth Hospital, Woodville, Australia

C. Russell, BA, BM BCh, FRACS
Central and Northern Adelaide Renal and Transplantation Service,
Royal Adelaide Hospital, Adelaide, Australia

J. Walsh, MD, FRACS
Discipline of Surgery, The Flinders University of South Australia, Adelaide, Australia

C. Jurisevic, MD, FRACS
Department of Surgery, Royal Adelaide Hospital, Adelaide, Australia

B.J. Coventry, BMBS, PhD, FRACS, FACS, FRSM
Discipline of Surgery, Royal Adelaide Hospital, University of Adelaide,
L5 Eleanor Harrald Building, North Terrace, 5000 Adelaide, SA, Australia
e-mail: brendon.coventry@adelaide.edu.au

B.J. Coventry (ed.), *Cardio-Thoracic, Vascular, Renal and Transplant Surgery,*
Surgery: Complications, Risks and Consequences,
DOI 10.1007/978-1-4471-5418-1_3, © Springer-Verlag London 2014

formation and **systemic sepsis**. **Multisystem failure** and **death** remain serious potential complications from vascular surgery and systemic infection.

Neural injuries are not infrequent potential problems associated with vascular surgery, because nerves commonly travel with vessels and are at risk of injury during dissection.

The risk of **bowel, bladder,** and **sexual dysfunction** increases with proximity to the pelvis and is almost exclusively associated with aortic and iliac surgery.

Positioning on the operating table has been associated with increased risk of **deep venous thrombosis** and **nerve palsies**, especially in prolonged procedures. **Limb ischemia, compartment syndrome, and ulnar** and **common peroneal nerve palsy** are recognized as potential complications, which should be checked for, as the patient's position may change during surgery.

Mortality associated with vascular procedures ranges from <0.1 % for simple procedures up to >80 % overall (30-day perioperative mortality) for individual urgent complex high-risk vascular procedures. In a study of 12,406 patients (1995–1999) undergoing abdominal aortic aneurysm repair, mortality varied from 4 % for elective repairs to 45 % for emergency (ruptured AAA) procedures. Variation of this type is well recognized and relatively common, depending on the underlying disease, type of procedure, and the extent of comorbidities, which needs to be taken into account when assessing risk or interpreting data.

This chapter therefore attempts to draw together in one place, the estimated overall frequencies of the complications associated with vascular disease, based on information obtained from the literature and experience. Not all patients are at risk of the full range of listed complications. It must be individualized for each patient and their disease process but represents a guide and summary of the attendant risks, complications, and consequences.

With these factors and facts in mind, the information given in this chapter must be appropriately and discernibly interpreted and used.

The **use of specialized units with standardized preoperative assessment, multidisciplinary input, and high-quality postoperative care** is essential to the success of complex vascular surgery overall and significantly reduces risk of complications or aid early detection, prompt intervention, and cost.

Important Note

It should be emphasized that the risks and frequencies that are given here *represent derived figures*. These *figures are best estimates of relative frequencies across most institutions*, not merely the highest-performing ones, and as such are often representative of a number of studies, which include different patients with differing comorbidities and different surgeons. In addition, the risks of complications in lower or higher risk patients may lie outside these estimated ranges, and individual clinical judgement is required as to the expected risks communicated to the patient, staff, or for other purposes. The range of risks is also derived from experience and the literature; while risks outside this range may exist, certain risks may be reduced or absent due to variations of procedures or surgical approaches. It is recognized that different patients, practitioners, institutions, regions, and countries may vary in their requirements and recommendations.

For complications related to other associated/additional surgery that may arise during arterial surgery, see the relevant volume and chapter, for example, Small Bowel Surgery Volume 4 or Thoracotomy (Chap. 8).

The authors would like to thank Professors Jack Collin, Peter Morris, and Dr Linda Hands, Oxford, United Kingdom, for their discussions and advice.

Diagnostic Angiography

Note: More complex angiographic procedures (including angioplasty, therapeutic embolization, stenting, and cardiac valve procedures) are associated with increased frequency of listed complications, risk of other complications, and often more specific complications (e.g., related to the body region, vessel disease, or procedure performed). Complication risk also varies with the urgency of the procedure, with emergency trauma-related procedures generally having higher overall risk.

Description

Local anesthetic is infiltrated into the region of the intended arterial puncture (usually the common femoral artery). Most procedures are performed under LA alone; however, sedation or general anesthesia may also be used. The underlying artery is punctured with a needle, through which a wire is passed, and then using a Seldinger technique a catheter is positioned in the vessel of interest. The aim is to inject a contrast agent while screening with digital subtraction to obtain images of the target vessel(s). Using a selection from a large variety of wires, catheters, and sheaths, the technique can be used to perform a range of procedures including radiocontrast dye injection, to position angioplasty balloons or stents, retrieve foreign bodies, deliver thrombolytic agents, or embolize bleeding vessels. Following completion of the procedure, the catheter or sheath is removed from the artery and the artery compressed to achieve hemostasis.

Anatomical Points

The common femoral artery begins where the external iliac artery passes under the inguinal ligament; note this is several centimeters superior to the flexural skin crease in the groin. Classically it has four branches (superficial circumflex iliac, superficial external pudendal, deep external pudendal, superficial epigastric), but their number and position is variable. The common femoral artery passes anterior to the femoral head, which is important as it provides a solid structure against which to compress the artery for hemostasis at the end of the procedure. The common femoral artery extends for approximately 5 cm before dividing into the superficial femoral and profunda femoris arteries. The origin of the profunda femoris may arise proximally even at the inguinal ligament or more distally. The origins and courses of vessels in the head, neck, upper limb, chest, abdomen, and pelvis can vary considerably, both anatomically and when affected by disease.

Perspective

See Table 3.1. Significant puncture site complications occur with a frequency of 0.1–1 %. Small hematomata are common, but rarely do they require surgical intervention. Large hematomata may lead to skin necrosis. Pseudoaneurysm and arteriovenous fistula formation are less common. Dissection also occurs with a frequency of 0.1–1 % and may occur at the puncture site or more distally from a catheter. These do not usually result in clinical complication especially if they are retrograde dissections but may lead to vessel occlusion. Embolization may occur due to air bubbles, thrombus formation on the catheter or from cholesterol embolization due to catheter manipulation in atheromatous vessels. This may lead to ischemia or blue-toe syndrome depending on the distal vascular bed (e.g., stroke, renal failure, gangrene) and the size of the embolized particles. Contrast-related complications include allergic reactions, which are only very rarely anaphylactic in nature, or contrast-induced nephropathy. Nephropathy can be avoided by careful checking of renal function pre-procedure, while limiting contrast dose and optimizing hydration. Contrast-related allergies can cause rash, nausea and vomiting, respiratory compromise, cardiac arrhythmia, hypotension, myocardial infarction, cardiac arrest, and death. Nephropathy can be avoided by good preoperative hydration and limiting contrast dose and by better awareness of renal status using preoperative renal function testing. Radiation burns are very rare. All complications are more common as the complexity of the intervention increases, and for groin procedures, related complications increase with larger sheath sizes. Bleeding risk is increased where thrombolytic agent infusions are used. Lymphocele or lymph leakage is usually minor.

Major Complications

The major risks include **bleeding, large hematoma formation, skin necrosis,** and **false aneurysm formation,** which may necessitate **further surgery. Distal ischemia** of a vascular bed is less common but may be devastating, depending on the location and underlying pathology, including **stroke, gut ischemia, bleeding** or **perforation,** and **limb ischemia** perhaps requiring **amputation. Severe allergic reactions,** including **anaphylaxis,** to radiographic contrast can occur and may rarely require resuscitation and ICU care. **Acute renal failure** may occur following renal arterial embolization or contrast agent-induced renal toxicity. **Thrombosis** or

Table 3.1 Angiography (excluding angioplasty and stenting): estimated frequency of complications, risks, and consequences

Complications, risks, and consequences	Estimated frequency
Most significant/serious complications	
Vascular complications	
Bleeding or hematoma formation	
Wound (small)	20–50 %
Wound (large)[a]	0.1–1 %
Graft associated (if graft is present)[a]	1–5 %
Vascular injury (femoral/popliteal artery or vein)[a]	0.1–1 %
Arterial wall dissection[a]	0.1–1 %
Embolization (thrombus, gas, or atheroma)[a]	0.1–1 %
Peripheral limb ischemia (trash foot/leg)[a]	0.1–1 %
Deep venous thrombosis/pulmonary embolus	0.1–1 %
Pseudoaneurysm (false aneurysm)[a]	0.1–1 %
Limb amputation[a]	<0.1 %
Arteriovenous fistula[a]	<0.1 %
Limb compartment syndrome (may necessitate fasciotomy)[a]	<0.1 %
Infection	
Wound[a]	<0.1 %
Systemic sepsis[a]	<0.1 %
Neural injury[a]	1–5 %
Sensory (ilioinguinal, femoral nerve/lat. cut. nerve thigh)	0.1–1 %
Motor (femoral)	0.1–1 %
Contrast-related complications (overall)	1–5 %
Allergic reactions (mild urticaria, mild asthma, itching)	1–5 %
Anaphylactic reactions	<0.1 %
Contrast-induced nephropathy	0.1–1 %
Rare significant/serious problems	
Organ ischemia (brain, abdominal)[a]	0.1–1 %
Gas gangrene or necrotizing fasciitis[a]	< 0.1 %
Cardiac events, respiratory failure, multisystem organ failure, death[a]	< 0.1 %
Less serious complications	
Skin necrosis or skin ulceration[a]	0.1–1 %
Seroma/lymphocele formation or lymphatic fluid leak	0.1–1 %
Limb edema (long-term swelling)[a]	<0.1 %
X-ray radiation burns[a]	<0.1 %
Blood transfusion[a]	0.1–1 %

NB: Many of these risks increase where interventions such as angioplasty, therapeutic embolization, stenting, and similar procedures are added to diagnostic angiography
[a]Dependent on underlying pathology, anatomy, experience, surgical technique, catheter sizes, and preferences

embolism often increases the relative risk of further complications. **Severe limb edema** is a very rare complication. In patients with vascular disease, the risk of **cardiorespiratory compromise** (e.g., myocardial infarction, cardiac failure,

Consent and Risk Reduction

Main Points to Explain

- Discomfort
- Bleeding*
- False aneurysm*
- Allergic reactions
- Distal embolization*
- Further surgery
- Risks without surgery

*Dependent on catheter size and site

cardiac arrhythmias) and embolic events is increased, which may rarely lead to **multisystem organ failure** and **death**. The frequency and range of the complications increase proportionately with the complexity of the angiographic intervention, and with groin procedures and larger catheter sheath sizes.

Temporal Artery Biopsy

Description

Local anesthesia or general anesthesia may be used. The aim is to expose and biopsy a part of the superficial temporal artery for diagnosis/exclusion of temporal arteritis. A preauricular incision is made in the hairline along the line of the artery to expose the temporal artery. A 4–7 cm segment is biopsied between clamps, inclusive of any pathological region if identifiable, and the ends are ligated with absorbable suture. The skin is closed.

Anatomical Points

The location of the temporal artery is relatively constant, but the branching and tortuosity may vary considerably, especially more distally at the hairline where the biopsy is usually performed. The superficial temporal artery lies superficial to the temporalis muscle fascia, but deep to the superficial fascia (which may be well developed at this site). The parietal branch can be given off early or later, and either the main trunk or parietal branch is usually chosen for the biopsy. The auriculotemporal nerve (branch of trigeminal V cranial n.) travels with the superficial temporal artery for much of its course and is at risk of injury.

Table 3.2 Temporal artery biopsy: estimated frequency of complications, risks, and consequences

Complications, risks, and consequences	Estimated frequency
Most significant/serious complications	
Infection	0.1–1 %
Bleeding and hematoma formation	0.1–1 %
Less serious complications	
Thrombosis	0.1–1 %
Failure to locate the temporal artery	0.1–1 %
Failure to sample the diseased arterial segment	5–20 %
Superficial temporal nerve injury (sensory loss)	1–5 %
Neuroma	0.1–1 %
Wound scarring (poor cosmesis)	1–5 %

[a]Dependent on underlying pathology, anatomy, surgical technique, and preferences

Perspective

See Table 3.2. Temporal artery biopsy is a small surgical procedure where most complications are relatively uncommon or less significant. However, **bleeding, hematoma formation, infection, failure to locate and biopsy the diseased artery,** and **nerve injury** are sometimes problematic.

Major Complications

The major complications are rare and are related to the wound itself, namely, **bleeding, hematoma formation,** and consequent **infection**, sometimes resulting in **wound dehiscence. Failure to locate and biopsy the diseased artery** may necessitate **repeat surgery** and inadvertent **auriculotemporal nerve injury** or even biopsy of it can occur, notably when obscured by bleeding from the vessel or its small branches, which can bleed profusely.

Consent and Risk Reduction

Main Points to Explain

- Discomfort
- Bleeding
- Failure to locate artery
- Failure to biopsy disease
- Nerve injury and numbness
- Infection
- Further surgery
- Risks without surgery

Arteriovenous Fistula Surgery

Description

Local anesthetic or local block is usually used. General anesthesia may be required for more extensive and revisional procedures. The aim is to create a superficial, straight segment of arterialized vein for hemodialysis access. The cephalic vein is the first choice and the anastomosis should be as distal as possible provided the artery and vein are of adequate caliber. It is important to ensure that the vein is patent, usually by flushing with heparinized saline. The cephalic vein is usually divided and sutured end-to-side to the radial artery via a longitudinal arteriotomy. Side-to-side or end-to-end anastomoses can also be performed. If performing an upper arm fistula, the same principles apply, but the incision in the artery should be small, so as to limit the risk of a "steal" phenomenon, particularly in the elderly or diabetic patient.

Anatomical Points

The first choice of vessels is the radial artery and cephalic vein in the forearm. The cutaneous branch of the radial nerve is in the vicinity and small branches may be inadvertently divided. If using the radial artery, it is important to ensure the presence of the ulnar, usually by Allen's test or duplex ultrasound if there is any doubt. Lack of a complete palmar arch may compromise vascularity of the hand. An upper arm brachiocephalic fistula is the next choice with other options being an ulnar-basilic forearm fistula, a transposed basilic vein to brachial artery in the upper arm, a saphenous loop in the thigh, or using prosthetic material to bridge between an artery and a vein. Prosthetic material currently remains the last choice for grafting. The brachial artery may have a high division such that the anastomosis at the elbow is onto either the radial or ulnar artery. It is important to assess the vein to ensure patency. Veins may not be present, e.g., upper arm cephalic, or may be damaged.

Perspective

See Table 3.3. The worst complications for the patient are either acute hand/limb ischemia or thrombosis of the fistula. Acute ischemia of the distal limb is extremely rare and is usually due to clot or spasm of the artery. It requires immediate exploration. Acute thrombosis of the fistula may be due to poor vessels, anastomotic technique, or hypotension. It should also be explored as soon as possible to try and salvage the fistula. A rare but important complication is acute ischemic neuritis of the median nerve. This *may* respond to immediate ligation of the fistula.

Table 3.3 Arteriovenous fistula surgery: estimated frequency of complications, risks, and consequences

Complications, risks, and consequences	Estimated frequency
Most significant/serious complications	
Infection (overall)[a]	1–5 %
Wound	1–5 %
Systemic sepsis	0.1–1 %
Bleeding or hematoma formation	1–5 %
Steal phenomenon/brachial fistula[a]	5–20 %
Acute fistula thrombosis[b]	1–5 %
Secondary problems	
Secondary patency	
1 year	70–80 %
5 year	50 %
Subacute bacterial endocarditis	0.1–1 %
Embolization	0.1–1 %
Fistula rupture	0.1–1 %
Rare significant/serious problems	
Fistula not usable[a] (anastomosis too small, peripheral vein previously damaged, subclavian vein stenosis from previous central venous lines)	0.1–1 %
Significant aneurysm formation[c]	0.1–1 %
Cardiac failure	0.1–1 %
Fistula thumb (blue hot painful thumb with varicose ulceration)[a] (notably with side-to-side anastomosis)	0.1–1 %
Acute ischemic neuritis of median nerve in upper arm fistula	<0.1 %
Acute ischemia (solitary supply; negative Allen's test)[a]	<0.1 %
Gas gangrene/necrotizing fasciitis	<0.1 %
Multisystem organ failure[a]	<0.1 %
Death[a]	<0.1 %
Less serious complications	
Numbness dorsum of thumb	1–5 %
Skin necrosis	0.1–1 %
Wound dehiscence	1–5 %
Delayed wound healing (including ulceration)	1–5 %
Wound scarring (poor cosmesis)[a]	1–5 %
Seroma/lymphocele formation	1–5 %
Residual pain/discomfort/neuralgia	1–5 %

[a]Dependent on underlying pathology, anatomy, surgical technique, and preferences
[b]Failure to develop the fistula and acute thrombosis are very operator dependent – this may depend on the patient population, whether only excellent vessels are used or whether attempts are made using less suitable vessels
[c]Virtually all fistulas will be aneurysmal once they have been needled. Significant aneurysm problems requiring repair are rare

Major Complications

Postoperative **acute fistula thrombosis** may be due to a stenosis in the vein, low blood pressure, or technical problems. **Acute loss of fistula function** requires immediate exploration. Postoperative **bleeding** can occlude the fistula from external pressure (often due to a slipped ligature on the distal end of the vein). **Steal phenomenon** is more common in upper arm fistulae, the elderly, and diabetics. It is important in brachial artery fistulae to limit the size of the arteriotomy – it should be <75 % of the proximal arterial diameter. **Stenoses** can develop at anastomotic sites, curves, and valves. **Revisional surgery** is often necessary at some point. Division of radial nerve branches may lead to **numbness** over the dorsum of the thumb. **Later secondary problems** include **shunt thrombosis, bacterial endocarditis, embolization,** and **fistula rupture. Infection** may occasionally be severe and lead to **dehiscence** and even **systemic sepsis**.

Consent and Risk Reduction

Main Points to Explain

- Discomfort
- Bleeding
- False aneurysm
- Fistula failure
- Distal ischemia
- Infection
- Further surgery
- Risks without surgery

Brachial Embolectomy (Including Graft Embolectomy)

Description

General or local anesthetic may be used. The aim is to gain entry to the brachial artery usually at the inferior cubital fossa, upper arm, or axilla to pass a balloon catheter proximally and distally beyond the embolus or thrombus to be able to draw embolic material retrogradely back through the arteriotomy to remove it and restore patency to the distal vessel(s). A vein patch may be needed to close the artery. An angiogram may be performed to ensure patency and infusion with a thrombolytic agent may be used. The arteriotomy and skin are then closed.

Anatomical Points

The site and extent of the embolus/thrombus will largely determine the site of arteriotomy and the vessels that need to be embolectomized. The arterial anatomy of the

Table 3.4 Brachial embolectomy: estimated frequency of complications, risks, and consequences

Complications, risks, and consequences	Estimated frequency
Most significant/serious complications	
Bleeding or hematoma formation	
Wound	5–20 %
Return to theater rate for evacuation of hematoma	1–5 %
Graft associated (if graft is present)[a]	1–5 %
Dissection of vessel wall and/or false aneurysm[a]	1–5 %
Re-thrombosis/blockage[a]	1–5 %
Further embolization[a] (thrombus or atheroma)	5–20 %
Rare significant/serious problems	
Infection	
Wound[a]	0.1–1 %
Systemic sepsis[a]	0.1–1 %
Neural injury[a]	0.1–1 %
Sensory (lateral cutaneous nerve of arm/forearm, brachial plexus)	
Motor (brachial plexus)	
Peripheral limb ischemia (trash hand/arm)[a]	0.1–1 %
Limb amputation[a]	0.1–1 %
Deep venous thrombosis/pulmonary embolus	0.1–1 %
Vascular injury (axillary/brachial artery or vein)[a]	0.1–1 %
Gas gangrene/necrotizing fasciitis[a]	<0.1 %
Limb compartment syndrome (may necessitate fasciotomy)[a]	<0.1 %
Less serious complications	
Skin ulceration[a]	0.1–1 %
Wound dehiscence	0.1–1 %
Seroma/lymphocele formation	1–5 %
Lymphatic fluid leak	1–5 %
Arm edema (long-term swelling)[a]	0.1–1 %
Wound scarring/deformity – poor cosmesis	0.1–1 %
Blood transfusion[a]	0.1–1 %
Wound drainage tube[a]	1–5 %

[a]Dependent on underlying pathology, anatomy, surgical technique, and preferences

larger vessels of the upper limb is relatively constant; however, the size of the embolectomy catheter in proportion to artery size will determine the distal extent of the embolectomy.

Perspective

See Table 3.4. Local wound problems, **hematoma, infection, and scarring,** are probably the most common complication of the arteriotomy and embolectomy surgery. **Nerve problems** are rare but can cause chronic pain on occasions. Severe complications are relatively rare but include **re-thrombosis/embolism, inability to**

remove the embolus, and amputation. Bleeding is a risk because all patients require postoperative anticoagulation to prevent further embolization. This risk is further increased when thrombolytic agent infusions are used.

Major Complications

The major risks are **bleeding, hematoma formation,** and **failure to remove the embolus,** which can result in **ischemia** and **amputation. Recurrence of thrombosis/embolus** can occur and increases the relative risk of further complications. **Severe arm edema** is a rare complication.

Consent and Risk Reduction

Main Points to Explain

- Discomfort
- Bleeding*
- False aneurysm*
- Further thromboembolism*
- Further surgery
- Risks without surgery

*Dependent on catheter size and site

Femoropopliteal Embolectomy (Including Graft Embolectomy)

Description

General or local anesthetic may be used. The aim is to gain entry to the femoropopliteal artery usually at the groin, but occasionally the mid-thigh or popliteal fossa, to pass a balloon catheter beyond the embolus or thrombus to be able to draw embolic material back through the arteriotomy to remove it and restore patency to the distal vessel(s). A vein patch may be needed to close the artery. An angiogram may be performed to ensure patency, and infusion with a thrombolytic agent may be used. The arteriotomy and skin are then closed.

Anatomical Points

The site and extent of the embolus/thrombus will largely determine the site of arteriotomy and the vessels that need to be embolectomized. The arterial anatomy

Table 3.5 Femoropopliteal embolectomy (including graft embolectomy): estimated frequency of complications, risks, and consequences

Complications, risks, and consequences	Estimated frequency
Most significant/serious complications	
Bleeding or hematoma formation	
Wound	1–5 %
Graft associated (if graft is present)[a]	1–5 %
Dissection of vessel wall and/or false aneurysm[a]	1–5 %
Re-thrombosis/blockage/embolization[a]	5–20 %
Vascular injury (femoral/popliteal artery or vein)[a]	0.1–1 %
Infection	
Wound[a]	5–20 %
Systemic sepsis[a]	0.1–1 %
Neural injury[a]	1–5 %
Sensory (ilioinguinal, femoral nerve/lat. cut. nerve thigh)	1–5 %
Motor (femoral)	0.1–1 %
Limb compartment syndrome (may necessitate fasciotomy)[a]	5–20 %
Limb amputation[a] (dependant on total ischemic time)	5–20 %
Acute renal failure	1–5 %
Cardiac complications (e.g., arrhythmias, failure, ischemic events)	1–5 %
Rare significant/serious problems	
Peripheral limb ischemia (trash foot/leg)[a]	0.1–1 %
Deep venous thrombosis/pulmonary embolus	0.1–1 %
Gas gangrene/necrotizing fasciitis[a]	<0.1 %
Less serious complications	
Skin ulceration[a]	0.1–1 %
Wound dehiscence	0.1–1 %
Seroma/lymphocele formation	1–5 %
Lymphatic fluid leak (esp. groin incisions)	1–5 %
Leg edema (long-term swelling)[a]	1–5 %
Wound scarring/deformity – poor cosmesis	0.1–1 %
Blood transfusion[a]	0.1–1 %
Wound drainage tube[a]	1–5 %

[a]Dependent on underlying pathology, anatomy, surgical technique, and preferences

of the larger vessels of the lower limb is relatively constant; however, the size of the embolectomy catheter in proportion to artery size will determine the distal extent of the embolectomy.

Perspective

See Table 3.5. Local wound problems, **hematoma, infection, and scarring,** are probably the most common complication of the arteriotomy and embolectomy surgery. **Nerve problems** are uncommon but can cause chronic pain on occasions. Severe complications are relatively rare but include **re-thrombosis/embolism, inability to remove the embolus, and amputation. Bleeding** risk is increased where thrombolytic agent infusions are used. **Lymphocele** or **lymph leakage** is not uncommon.

Major Complications

The major risks are **bleeding** and **hematoma formation** and **failure to remove the embolus,** which can result in **ischemia** and **amputation. Recurrence of thrombosis/embolus** can occur and increases the relative risk of further complications. **Severe leg edema** is a rare complication.

> **Consent and Risk Reduction**
>
> **Main Points to Explain**
>
> - Discomfort
> - Bleeding*
> - False aneurysm*
> - Further thromboembolism*
> - Further surgery
> - Risks without surgery
>
> *Dependent on catheter size and site

Mesenteric Arterial Embolectomy

Description

General anesthetic is used. The aim is to gain entry to the superior mesenteric, celiac, or very rarely inferior mesenteric artery usually during laparotomy to pass a balloon catheter proximally and distally beyond the embolus or thrombus to be able to draw embolic material back through the arteriotomy to remove it and restore patency to the distal vessel(s) and bowel. A vein patch may be needed to close the artery. An angiogram may be performed to ensure patency and infusion with a thrombolytic agent may be used. The arteriotomy and skin are then closed.

Anatomical Points

The site and extent of the embolus/thrombus will largely determine the site of arteriotomy and the vessels that need to be embolectomized. The arterial anatomy of the larger vessels of the mesenteric circulation is relatively constant, but the smaller vessels may vary considerably; however the size of the embolectomy catheter in proportion to artery size will determine the distal extent of the embolectomy. Mesenteric arteries tend to be thinner walled than systemic vessels and are more fragile, being liable to rupture. The anatomy of the vascular supply may be significantly altered by atheroma, even with occlusion and reversal of flow with blood supply coming from other vascular channels.

Perspective

See Table 3.6. This condition often initially presents with vague initial symptoms and signs, and delayed diagnosis is common, such that if established gut ischemia is present with sepsis, mortality is likely. When diagnosed expediently, the clinical picture is often of severe abdominal pain with minimal clinical signs, atrial

Table 3.6 Mesenteric arterial embolectomy: estimated frequency of complications, risks, and consequences

Complications, risks, and consequences	Estimated frequency
Most significant/serious complications	
Bleeding or hematoma formation	
Wound	1–5 %
Graft associated (if graft is present)[a]	1–5 %
Dissection of vessel wall and/or false aneurysm[a]	1–5 %
Re-thrombosis/blockage[a]	1–5 %
Further embolization[a] (thrombus or atheroma)	5–20 %
Vascular injury (mesenteric/femoral/popliteal artery or vein)[a]	1–5 %
Graft dehiscence/leakage/rupture[a]	1–5 %
Infection	
Wound[a]	0.1–1 %
Systemic sepsis[a]	5–20 %
Colonic ischemia/necrosis[a]	50–80 %
Myocardial impairment/failure[a]	5–20 %
Pulmonary impairment/failure[a]	5–20 %
Renal impairment/failure[a]	5–20 %
Gastrointestinal hemorrhage (ischemic gut)[a]	1–5 %
Abdominal compartment syndrome (may necessitate re-laparotomy)[a]	1–5 %
Small bowel obstruction (adhesions or ischemia)[a]	1–5 %
Trash kidney[a]	1–5 %
Multisystem failure (renal, pulmonary, cardiac failure)[a]	5–20 %
Death[a]	>80 %
Rare significant/serious problems	
Gut injury/perforation (traumatic)[a]	0.1–1 %

(continued)

Table 3.6 (continued)

Complications, risks, and consequences	Estimated frequency
Neural injury[a]	0.1–1 %
Sensory (subcostal, ilioinguinal, iliohypogastric)	
Motor (lumbosacral plexus)	
Pancreatitis	0.1–1 %
Peripheral limb ischemia (trash foot/leg)[a]	0.1–1 %
Deep venous thrombosis/pulmonary embolus	0.1–1 %
Gas gangrene/necrotizing fasciitis[a]	<0.1 %
Limb compartment syndrome (may necessitate fasciotomy)[a]	<0.1 %
Less serious complications	
Skin ulceration[a]	0.1–1 %
Wound dehiscence	0.1–1 %
Lymphatic fluid leak/chylous ascites/fistula[a]	1–5 %
Paralytic ileus	50–80 %
Leg edema (long-term swelling)[a]	0.1–1 %
Orchitis/testicular atrophy[a]	0.1–1 %
Wound scarring/deformity – poor cosmesis	0.1–1 %
Incisional hernia formation (delayed heavy lifting or straining)	0.1–1 %
Blood transfusion[a]	0.1–1 %
Wound drainage tube[a]	1–5 %

[a]Dependent on underlying pathology, anatomy, surgical technique, and preferences

fibrillation and episodes of recurrent embolization. **Multisystem failure** and **death** is the usual outcome due to the fact that most patients are elderly with significant comorbidities and that the diagnosis is often made late. Local wound problems, **hematoma, infection, and scarring,** are probably the most common complications of abdominal arteriotomy and embolectomy surgery. **Nerve problems** are uncommon but can cause chronic pain on occasions. Severe complications are relatively rare but include **re-thrombosis/embolism, inability to remove the embolus, and mesenteric ischemia.** Mesenteric ischemia may cause **serious bowel complications,** with or without the further surgery. **Bleeding** risk is increased where thrombolytic agent infusions are used.

Major Complications

The major risks are **bleeding, hematoma formation,** and **failure to remove the embolus,** which can result in **ischemia** and **mesenteric ischemia. Bowel resection** may be required. **Recurrence of thrombosis/embolus** can occur and increases the relative risk of further complications. **False aneurysm** can occur at the femoral or brachial puncture site(s). **Bleeding, perforation, and stenosis of the bowel** may occur, requiring **further surgery. Multisystem organ failure** is related closely to preexisting ischemic time, comorbidities, and age, often resulting in **death**. Many of the major complications arise from the underlying disease state and comorbidities with the typical patient being elderly, having an embolic history, cardiac arrhythmias (usually AF), with severe abdominal pain and few signs, presenting late with established gut ischemia.

Consent and Risk Reduction

Main Points to Explain

- Discomfort
- Bleeding*
- False aneurysm*
- Further thromboembolism*
- Further surgery
- Risks without surgery

*Dependent on catheter size and site

Carotid Endarterectomy

Description

General or local anesthetic may be used. The aim is to expose the carotid artery(s) to perform an arteriotomy to remove atheromatous plaque, debris, and thrombus from the luminal aspect to improve flow through the carotid vessels. The carotid vessels are clamped above and below the obstructing stenosis and the arteriotomy performed between. The carotid blood flow may be bypassed around the operative site with the use of a shunt, intraoperatively, to preserve perfusion of the brain and other distal tissues. The arteriotomy is frequently closed with a vein patch and continuous monofilament sutures. The skin is often closed with continuous absorbable suture.

Anatomical Points

The carotid arterial anatomy is relatively constant with the carotid bifurcation at approximately hyoid cartilage/C3 vertebral level. The extent, nature, and degree of the carotid stenosis usually dictate the site and surgical approach. The arterial anatomy can also be altered by the atherosclerotic disease process to some degree, affecting the vascular tortuosity.

Perspective

See Table 3.7. Local wound problems, **hematoma, infection, and scarring**, are probably the most common complications of carotid arterial surgery. **Nerve problems** (especially neck and ear numbness from injury to the cervical plexus) are not uncommon but can cause chronic pain on occasions. Permanent clinically significant cranial nerve injuries are rare. Severe complications include **TIAs, stroke, myocardial infarction,** and **death** but fortunately are relatively uncommon.

Major Complications

The major risks are **acute bleeding** and **hematoma formation** which may produce **life-threatening respiratory obstruction,** requiring immediate surgical drainage to relieve the pressure. **Embolization or thrombosis** can result in **TIAs, RINDs, and stroke** which are significant sequelae and potentially catastrophic. Intimal hyperplasia and atheroma causing **carotid restenosis** is a significant late problem. **False aneurysm** is another complication of surgery to the vessel wall in the medium to late term. Subtle cerebral injuries causing psychological changes are relatively common and are determined by how closely examinations are performed. Some changes may represent those present but missed in the preoperative assessment. **Injury to the facial nerve** can be permanent and cause permanent facial paralysis, particularly affecting the corner of the mouth causing dribbling. Further surgery may be required for correction of this. **Numbness of the neck** is occasionally a significant problem for some patients, especially with shaving or application of cosmetics. **Pneumothorax** and **lymphatic (chylous) leak** are extremely rare but can occur with low cervical dissections. **Lymphatic sinuses** are extremely rare, but **suture granulomas** can be troublesome and may require excision. **Wound scarring and deformity** are rarely a problem but may require revision surgery.

Consent and Risk Reduction

Main Points to Explain

- Discomfort
- Bleeding
- False aneurysm
- Stroke
- Carotid restenosis
- Infection
- Further surgery
- Risks without surgery

Table 3.7 Carotid endarterectomy: estimated frequency of complications, risks, and consequences

Complications, risks, and consequences	Estimated frequency
Most significant/serious complications	
Infection (overall)	1–5 %
Wound	0.1–1 %
Graft associated	0.1–1 %
Systemic sepsis	0.1–1 %
Bleeding or hematoma formation – overall	1–5 %
Early: wound/graft associated/false aneurysm	1–5 %
Late: graft failure tear dissection, etc.	0.1–1 %
Vessel/graft thrombosis/blockage	0.1–1 %
Carotid restenosis (intimal hyperplasia or atheroma)	5–20 %
Cerebral ischemia/hemorrhage/thrombosis (CVA, TIA, RIND)[a]	1–5 %
Myocardial impairment/failure[a]	1–5 %
Pulmonary impairment/failure[a]	1–5 %
Neural injury (paresthesia and/or muscle weakness)[a]	
Sensory (overall)	>80 %
Cervical plexus – neck/chest/facial numbness	>80 %
Lingual V – tongue numbness, sympathetic Horner's syndrome	0.1–1 %
Motor (overall)	5–20 %
Neuropraxia (temporary)	5–20 %
Nerve division (permanent)	0.1–1 %
(including facial VII, weakness; hypoglossal XII, tongue weakness; accessory XI, shoulder weakness; vagus X, voice changes; glossopharyngeal IX, swallowing difficulty; phrenic nerve injury, diaphragmatic paralysis)	
Death	1–5 %
Rare significant/serious problems	
Acute respiratory obstruction	0.1–1 %
Renal impairment/failure	0.1–1 %
Multisystem failure (renal, pulmonary, cardiac failure)	0.1–1 %
Deep venous thrombosis/pulmonary embolus	0.1–1 %
Epilepsy[a] (LA and hypoperfusion)	0.1–1 %
Pneumothorax[a]	0.1–1 %
False aneurysm formation	<0.1 %
First bite syndrome	<0.1 %
Less serious complications	
Skin ulceration	0.1–1 %
Psychological changes[a] (often subtle)	20–50 %
Seroma/lymphocele/chylous/lymphatic fluid leakage/fistula (right lymphatic or thoracic duct injury)[a]	0.1–1 %
Facial/neck swelling	5–20 %
Hyperesthesia	1–5 %
Blood transfusion	0.1–1 %
Wound dehiscence	0.1–1 %
Wound scarring/deformity (poor cosmesis)	0.1–1 %
Wound drain tube[a]	5–20 %

[a]Dependent on underlying pathology, anatomy, surgical technique, and preferences

Femoropopliteal Bypass Surgery (Including Femoro-tibial, Femoro-distal Bypass Surgery, and Femoro-femoral Crossover Graft Surgery)

Description

General anesthetic is usually used, but spinal/epidural anesthesia can be used. The aim is to bypass the obstructing lesion(s) in the femoral or popliteal artery. If iliac obstruction is present, a femoro-femoral crossover graft from the patent contralateral femoral or iliac artery may be required. Vein is currently the preferred conduit, usually using ipsilateral long saphenous vein (LSV), but synthetic graft material can be used. Vertical incisions are generally made in the groin and lower thigh/popliteal fossa or more distally for access as required according to the site of obstruction and the relatively normal caliber vessels for anastomosis.

Anatomical Points

The iliac and femoral arteries are relatively constant; however, the profunda femoris artery, the muscular perforators, and the location of division of the popliteal artery into its branches (anterior, posterior tibial and peroneal) are moderately variable. This latter division may occur anywhere within the popliteal fossa or below, and each branch leaves the artery at different levels. Angiography should usually map the divisions adequately. Pathology may cause stenosis, absence, and differing collateral circulation, which may alter anatomy significantly.

Perspective

See Table 3.8. Local wound problems, **hematoma, infection, and scarring,** are probably the most common complication of the femoral bypass graft surgery. **Graft infection** is about 3 times greater for prosthetic (Dacron; PTFE) grafts than for autologous saphenous vein grafts. If graft infection occurs, occlusion rates, amputation rates, and mortality are significantly increased. **Nerve problems** are not uncommon and can cause chronic pain on occasions. Severe complications increase with time from surgery and include **thrombosis/embolism,** lower limb **distal ischemia re-operative bypass surgery,** and **amputation. Bleeding** risk is increased where thrombolytic agent infusions are used. **Lymphocele** or **lymph leakage** is not uncommon. **Graft occlusion, recurrent ischemia,** and **groin hernia formation,** often prevascular, are common later events with this surgery. Amputation risk increases in proportion to the extent of underlying vascular obstruction.

Table 3.8 Femoropopliteal (–tibial) bypass surgery: estimated frequency of complications, risks, and consequences

Complications, risks, and consequences	Estimated frequency
Most significant/serious complications	
Bleeding or hematoma formation	
Wound	1–5 %
Graft dehiscence/leakage/rupture (early)[a] (including dissection of vessel wall; false aneurysm)	1–5 %
Late delayed bleeding (graft erosion)	0.1–1 %
Femoro-cutaneous fistula	<0.1 %
Early graft thrombosis/blockage[a]	1–5 %
Late graft failure (tearing, dissection, etc.)[a]	0.1–1 %
Embolization[a] (thrombus or atheroma)	1–5 %
Arteriovenous fistula (in situ saphenous vein bypass grafts)	1–5 %
Limb amputation (short term)[a]	
Claudicants	0.1–1 %
Critical limb ischemia	1–5 %
Limb amputation (late)[a]	
Claudicants	1–5 %
Critical limb ischemia	5–20 %
Infection	
Wound[a]	5–20 %
Graft associated[a]	0.1–1 %
Systemic sepsis[a]	0.1–1 %
Wound dehiscence	1–5 %
Seroma/lymphocele formation or lymphatic fluid leak	5–20 %
Myocardial impairment/infarction/failure[a]	1–5 %
Cerebral ischemia/hemorrhage/thrombosis (CVA, TIA, RIND)[a]	1–5 %
Neural injury[a] (overall)	1–5 %
Sensory (femoral nerve/lat. cut. nerve thigh/sciatic/saphenous)	
Motor (femoral)	
Death[a]	1–5 %
Rare significant/serious problems	
Limb compartment syndrome (may necessitate fasciotomy)[a]	<0.1 %
Vascular injury (femoral/popliteal artery or vein)[a]	0.1–1 %
Peripheral limb ischemia (trash foot/leg)[a]	0.1–1 %
Deep venous thrombosis/pulmonary embolus	0.1–1 %
Gas gangrene/necrotizing fasciitis[a]	0.1 %
Less serious complications	
Skin ulceration[a]	0.1–1 %
Femoral (or prevascular or inguinal) hernia (late)[a]	1–5 %
Leg edema (long-term swelling)[a] (rarely severe)	5–20 %
Wound scarring/deformity – poor cosmesis	0.1–1 %
Blood transfusion[a]	0.1–1 %
Wound drainage tube[a]	1–5 %

[a]Dependent on underlying pathology, anatomy, surgical technique, comorbidities, and preferences

Major Complications

The major risks are **intraoperative** and **postoperative bleeding** and **hematoma formation, sometimes resulting in wound infection**. Rarely, graft infection may result in catastrophic **graft rupture** and **acute hemorrhage**. **Graft infection** may require graft removal. Acute or chronic **graft thrombosis** may occur and can result in **ischemia, ulceration, re-operative bypass surgery,** and **amputation. Loss of patency** typically occurs as time progresses. **Amputation** risk increases as a function of vascular disease severity and time. **Severe leg edema** is rarely severe and may be assisted by stockings. **Lymphoceles** are usually self-limited but sometimes requiring repeated drainage and may predispose to infection. **Hernia formation** is typically prevascular and may occasionally result in **bowel obstruction** if untreated surgically. **Nerve injury** is rarely severe, but both femoral sensory and motor nerve branches are at risk. **Necrotizing fasciitis** is an extremely rare but devastating complication with a high mortality.

Consent and Risk Reduction

Main Points to Explain

- Discomfort
- Bleeding*
- False aneurysm*
- Distal embolization*
- Limb amputation*
- Further surgery*
- Risks without surgery

*Dependent on pathology, type of graft, and site

Abdominal Aortic Aneurysm Repair: Elective Aortic Aneurysm Repair (Including Aorto-bifemoral and Aortoiliac Graft Repairs)

Description

General anesthetic is used with muscle relaxation. A midline or transverse incision may be used. The aim is to expose the abdominal aorta and iliac vessels (if required) and obtain control of the aorta with placement of a large vascular clamp above the abdominal aortic aneurysm and also below it, usually across the iliac arteries. The aorta is typically incised longitudinally to expose the luminal contents of atheroma, calcification, and blood clot, which are extracted. The lumbar arteries and inferior mesenteric artery are then oversewn. The native adventitia and some media are typically preserved and the synthetic graft (e.g., Dacron or PTFE) is cut to length, inserted, and sutured in place proximally and distally. The graft is tested and the clamps slowly released to reperfuse the lower limbs and organs. The abdominal wall and skin is closed.

Anatomical Points

The normal aorta is constant in location being slightly to the left of midline; however, the anatomy may be highly distorted due to aneurysm formation and branch points may be greatly disparate from the normal anatomical situation. The renal, mesenteric, gonadal, and iliac vessels may be rendered tortuous and asymmetrical, requiring careful identification. Lumbar vessels are often variable in location and number and may cause troublesome bleeding during the repair, often requiring underrun suturing. Venous duplication or anomalies occur in some 5 % of patients, increasing the risk of injury during aortic clamping and dissection. The left renal vein is usually anterior to the aorta but may be posterior or even circum-aortic, where it may be injured. The aortic bifurcation may be at a slightly higher level in some individuals than others, and the anatomy may be altered by ectasia, tortuosity, or the aneurysmal dilatation (fusiform or saccular). Fusiform aneurysms may extend into the iliac vessels, altering anatomy and the surgical difficulty. The sites of the spinal blood supply (arteries of Adamkiewicz; T1 and T11) are variable and occlusion may cause spinal ischemia and paralysis.

Perspective

See Table 3.9. Despite the major nature of this surgery, local wound problems, **hematoma, infection, and scarring,** are probably the most common complications of the abdominal aortic aneurysm surgery. **Myocardial infarction** is a serious

Table 3.9 Elective abdominal aortic/iliac aneurysm repair: estimated frequency of complications, risks, and consequences

Complications, risks, and consequences	Estimated frequency
Most significant/serious complications	
Infection (overall)	5–20 %
Wound	1–5 %
Intra-abdominal	1–5 %
Graft associated	1–5 %
Systemic sepsis	1–5 %
Bleeding or hematoma formation	
Wound	1–5 %
Graft associated	1–5 %
Late graft failure (dissection, false aneurysm, prosthesis loosening, etc.)	1–5 %
Late events (aorto-cutaneous fistula, aorto-caval fistula, etc.)	<0.1 %
Graft thrombosis/blockage	0.1–1 %
Direct vascular injury (iliac/renal/mesenteric/femoral artery or vein)	0.1–1 %

(continued)

Table 3.9 (continued)

Complications, risks, and consequences	Estimated frequency
Embolization (thrombus/atheroma)	1–5 %
Peripheral limb ischemia (trash foot/leg)	1–5 %
Cerebral ischemia/hemorrhage/thrombosis (CVA, TIA, RIND)[a]	1–5 %
Mesenteric/colonic ischemia/necrosis[a]	1–5 %
Sexual dysfunction, impotence[b]	5–20 %
Small bowel obstruction (adhesions)	1–5 %
Renal impairment/failure	1–5 %
Myocardial impairment/infarction/failure	1–5 %
Pulmonary impairment/failure	1–5 %
Multisystem failure (renal, pulmonary, cardiac failure)	1–5 %
Death	5–20 %
Rare significant/serious problems	
Deep venous thrombosis/pulmonary embolus	0.1–1 %
Gut injury/perforation	0.1–1 %
Wound dehiscence	0.1–1 %
Paralysis and paraplegia (spinal cord ischemia ~ 1:200 straight; 1:100 ABF)	0.1–1 %
Ureteric injury	0.1–1 %
Pancreatitis/pancreatic cyst/fistula	0.1–1 %
Neural injury	
Sensory (sciatic, ilioinguinal, femoral nerve/lat. cut. nerve thigh)	0.1–1 %
Motor (sciatic, femoral)	0.1–1 %
Coagulopathy (DIC/consumption)	0.1–1 %
[a]"Trash" kidney	0.1–1 %
Abdominal compartment syndrome	0.1–1 %
Gastrointestinal hemorrhage (aorto-enteric fistula or ischemic gut)	< 0.1 %
Gas gangrene/necrotizing fasciitis[a]	< 0.1 %
Less serious complications	
Skin ulceration	0.1–1 %
Paralytic ileus	50–80 %
Femoral (or prevascular or inguinal) hernia (late aortoiliac or bifemoral aneurysm)	0.1–1 %
Psychological changes[a] (often subtle)	5–20 %
Seroma/lymphocele formation or lymphatic fluid leak[c]	1–5 %
Lymphatic ascites/chylous ascites/fistula	0.1–1 %
Hyperbilirubinemia (unconjugated/thrombus related)	0.1–1 %
[a]Orchitis/testicular atrophy	<0.1 %
Leg edema swelling	1–5 %
Incisional hernia formation (delayed heavy lifting or straining)	1–5 %
Wound scarring/deformity – poor cosmesis	1–5 %
Blood transfusion[a]	20–50 %
Wound drain[a] (particularly for ABF grafts)	50–80 %

ABF aorto-bifemoral, *RIND* reversible ischemic neurological deficit, *TIA* transient ischemic attack, *CVA* cerebrovascular accident
[a]Dependent on underlying pathology, anatomy, surgical technique, and preferences
[b]Impotence may be present preoperatively and should be determined before surgery
[c]If femoral or distal iliac arteries are exposed

complication of aortic aneurysm surgery with about a 3 % perioperative mortality and 5 % late mortality rate, with ~76 % alive at 5 years. **Nerve problems** are not uncommon, mainly of the abdominal wall, but are usually minor only causing chronic pain on occasions. Severe complications include **bleeding**, sometimes due to tearing of the calcified aorta during suturing or postoperatively at the anastomosis or due to lumbar vessels. **Mesenteric ischemia** due to low perfusion intraoperatively may cause **serious bowel complications,** with or without the further surgery. **Reperfusion injury** due to release of the clamps after a period of intraoperative ischemia to the lower body may result in acidosis, release of products of ischemia, and **hypotensive shock. Acute renal failure** due to reduced renal blood flow intraoperatively may occur and is more common with aneurysms extending above the renal arteries and is associated with increased mortality. **Renal dialysis** is required for renal failure in 1–5 % of cases. **Late thrombosis** of the graft can cause **distal ischemia** and/or **embolism**, including **mesenteric ischemia. Cardiac failure** may occur on release of the aortic cross-clamp and severe **pulmonary edema** may result. **Respiratory infections** are not uncommon, sometimes progressing to **pneumonia** and **adult respiratory distress syndrome** after prolonged surgery or previous respiratory compromise, including smoking. **Multisystem failure** is not uncommon particularly in elderly patients with significant comorbidities. **Coagulopathy** is not uncommon when multisystem failure becomes established. **Lymphocele** or **lymph leakage** is not uncommon but is rarely a clinical problem. **Abdominal hernia formation** is not uncommon, sometimes developing years after surgery, and is associated with surgical wound infection. Embolism of debris to limbs or organs may cause irreversible ischemia causing **trash foot, limb or digit amputation**, or **organ ischemia** and is another mechanism of organ failure (e.g., renal, cardiac, or gut complications). **Sexual dysfunction** may occur in both sexes but is less well documented in females.

Major Complications

The main serious complications of aortic aneurysm surgery result from bleeding, infection, or ischemia. In general aorto-bifemoral/biiliac repairs are associated with higher complication rates. Major **intraoperative** risks include serious **acute bleeding, cardiac failure,** and ischemia of limbs or organs, which can result in **circulatory collapse** when the aortic clamps are released at the procedure completion. Risk of **on-table death** is overall less than for emergency aortic repair procedures.

Postoperatively, there are considerable risks also mainly from **postoperative bleeding** and **hematoma formation**, sometimes resulting in **wound infection**. Rarely, **graft infection** may result in catastrophic **graft rupture** and **acute hemorrhage.** Graft infection may require graft removal and/or **re-operative bypass surgery**. Acute or chronic **graft thrombosis** may occur and can result in **ischemia, leg ulceration,** and even **limb/digit amputation. Loss of patency** can occur due to further disease at the anastomoses. **Severe leg edema** is a rare complication and may be assisted by stockings. **Sexual dysfunction** may occur due to inadvertent disruption of autonomic nerves; it may also predate surgery due to neurovascular disease. **Lymphoceles** are usually self-limited but sometimes require drainage and may predispose to infection. **Hernia formation** may occasionally result in **bowel obstruction** and require surgical repair. **Nerve injury** is rarely severe. **Aorto-enteric fistula** is a rare but catastrophic late complication, associated with acute melena, hematemesis, and/or severe hypotension. **Necrotizing fasciitis** is an extremely rare but devastating complication with a high mortality. **Renal failure** may require dialysis**, respiratory failure and ARDS** typically require prolonged ventilation, and **cardiac failure** may require inotropic and even pacemaker support. **Mesenteric ischemia** may require **bowel resection**. **GI bleeding, perforation, and stenosis of the bowel** may occur, requiring **further surgery**. **Multisystem organ failure** is a severe and often lethal complication related closely to preexisting pathology, comorbidities, and age.

Consent and Risk Reduction

Main Points to Explain

- Pain
- Bleeding*
- Infection*
- Distal embolization*
- Organ failure
- ICU care
- Further surgery
- Risks without surgery
- Death

*Dependent on pathology, graft, and site

Abdominal Aortic Aneurysm Repair: Emergency Aortic Aneurysm Repair (Including Aorto-bifemoral and Aortoiliac Graft Repairs)

Description

General anesthetic is used with muscle relaxation. A midline or transverse incision may be used. The aim is to rapidly expose the abdominal aorta, and iliac vessels (if required), and obtain control of the aorta with placement of a large vascular clamp above the abdominal aortic aneurysm and also below it, either across the very distal aorta or iliac arteries. Proximal control of the aorta may need to be achieved at the supra-coeliac level. Hematoma typically obscures the aorta and impedes easy access. The aorta is usually incised longitudinally to expose the luminal contents of atheroma, calcification, and blood clot, which is extracted. The native adventitia and some media are typically preserved and the synthetic graft (e.g., Dacron or PTFE) is cut to length, inserted, and sutured in place proximally and distally. The graft is tested and the clamps slowly released to reperfuse the lower limbs and organs. The abdominal wall and skin is closed.

Anatomical Points

The normal aorta is constant in location being slightly to the left of midline; however, the anatomy may be highly distorted due to aneurysm formation and branch points may be greatly disparate from the normal anatomical situation. The renal, mesenteric, gonadal, and iliac vessels may be rendered tortuous and asymmetrical, requiring careful identification. Lumbar vessels are often variable in location and number and may cause troublesome bleeding during the repair, often requiring underrun suturing. In the emergency setting hematoma from the leaking aneurysm may obscure and distort the anatomy significantly, increasing risk of vascular and neural injury. Venous duplication or anomalies occur in some 5 % of patients, increasing the risk of injury during aortic clamping and dissection. The left renal vein is usually anterior to the aorta but may be posterior (or rarely around), where it may be more easily injured. The aortic bifurcation may be at a slightly higher level in some individuals than others, and the anatomy may be altered by ectasia, tortuosity, or the aneurysmal dilatation (fusiform or saccular). Fusiform aneurysms may extend into the iliac vessels, altering anatomy and the surgical difficulty. The sites of the spinal blood supply (arteries of Adamkiewicz; T1 and T11) are variable and occlusion may cause spinal ischemia and paralysis.

Perspective

See Table 3.10. Overall, *emergency* aortic aneurysm repair carries much higher risks than equivalent elective repair, principally due to acute hemorrhage, hypotension, and ischemia. In general aorto-bifemoral/biiliac repairs are associated with higher complication rates. The risk of multisystem failure is notably higher. **Nerve**

Table 3.10 Emergency abdominal aortic/iliac aneurysm repair: estimated frequency of complications, risks, and consequences

Complications, risks, and consequences	Estimated frequency
Most significant/serious complications	
Infection (overall)	5–20 %
Wound	1–5 %
Intra-abdominal	1–5 %
Graft associated	1–5 %
Systemic sepsis	1–5 %

(continued)

Table 3.10 (continued)

Complications, risks, and consequences	Estimated frequency
Bleeding or hematoma formation	
Wound	1–5 %
Graft associated	1–5 %
False aneurysm	1–5 %
Late graft failure (dissection, false aneurysm, prosthesis loosening, etc.)	1–5 %
Late events (aorto-cutaneous fistula, aorto-caval fistula, etc.)	<0.1 %
Graft thrombosis/blockage/embolization	1–5 %
Direct vascular injury (iliac/renal/mesenteric/femoral artery or vein)	1–5 %
Deep venous thrombosis/pulmonary embolus	1–5 %
Peripheral limb ischemia ("trash" foot/leg)	5–20 %
Mesenteric/colonic ischemia/necrosis[a]	5–20 %
Sexual dysfunction/impotence[b]	5–20 %
Renal impairment/failure (including renal arterial/venous injury, hypoperfusion, or sepsis)	5–20 %
Myocardial impairment/infarction/failure	5–20 %
Pulmonary impairment/failure	5–20 %
Cerebral ischemia/hemorrhage/thrombosis (CVA, TIA, RIND)[a]	1–5 %
Paralysis and paraplegia (spinal cord ischemia ~ 1:100 straight; 1:50 ABF)	1–5 %
Coagulopathy (DIC/consumption)	1–5 %
Abdominal compartment syndrome	1–5 %
Small bowel obstruction (adhesions)	1–5 %
Multisystem failure (renal, pulmonary, cardiac failure)	20–50 %
Death	20–50 %
Rare significant/serious problems	
Neural injury[c]	
Sensory (sciatic, ilioinguinal, femoral nerve/lat. cut. nerve thigh)	0.1–1 %
Motor (sciatic, femoral)	0.1–1 %
Gut injury/perforation (duodenal, gastric, small bowel, colonic)	0.1–1 %
Ureteric injury	0.1–1 %
Pancreatitis/pancreatic cyst/fistula	0.1–1 %
Limb compartment syndrome (may necessitate fasciotomy)	0.1–1 %
"Trash'" kidney[a]	0.1–1 %
Gas gangrene/necrotizing fasciitis	<0.1 %
Gastrointestinal hemorrhage (aorto-enteric fistula or ischemic gut)	<0.1 %
Less serious complications	
Skin ulceration	0.1–1 %
Chylous ascites/fistula	0.1–1 %
Paralytic ileus	50–80 %
Psychological changes[a] (often subtle)	5–20 %
Seroma/lymphocele formation/lymphatic fluid leak/lymphatic ascites[a]	1–5 %
[a]Orchitis/testicular atrophy	1–5 %

Table 3.10 (continued)

Complications, risks, and consequences	Estimated frequency
Femoral (or prevascular or inguinal) hernia (late aortoiliac or bifemoral aneurysm)	0.1–1 %
Hyperbilirubinemia (unconjugated/thrombus related)	1–5 %
Leg edema swelling	1–5 %
Incisional hernia formation (delayed heavy lifting or straining)	1–5 %
Wound scarring/deformity – poor cosmesis	1–5 %
Blood transfusion[a]	>80 %
Wound dehiscence	1–5 %
Wound drain[a]	5–20 %

ABF aorto-bifemoral, *RIND* reversible ischemic neurological deficit, *TIA* transient ischemic attack, *CVA* cerebrovascular accident

[a]Dependent on underlying pathology, anatomy, surgical technique, and preferences

[b]Impotence may be present preoperatively and should be determined before surgery

[c]If femoral or distal iliac arteries are exposed

problems are not uncommon, mainly of the abdominal wall, but are usually minor only causing chronic pain on occasions. Severe complications include **bleeding**, sometimes due to tearing of the calcified aorta during suturing or postoperatively at the anastomosis or due to lumbar vessels. **Mesenteric ischemia** is reported to occur in up to 60 % of emergency repair cases due to low perfusion intraoperatively, which may cause **serious bowel complications,** with or without the further surgery. **Reperfusion injury** due to release of the clamps after a period of intraoperative ischemia to the lower body may result in acidosis, release of products of ischemia, and **hypotensive shock. Acute renal failure** due to reduced renal blood flow intraoperatively may occur and is more common with ruptured aneurysms (over 70 % cases) and those extending above the renal arteries. It is associated with an increased mortality of over 50 %. Renal failure may require **renal dialysis. Late thrombosis** of the graft can cause **distal ischemia** and/or **embolism**, including **mesenteric ischemia. Cardiac failure** may occur on release of the aortic cross-clamp, and severe **pulmonary edema** may result. **Respiratory infections** are not uncommon, sometimes progressing to **pneumonia** and **adult respiratory distress syndrome** after prolonged surgery or previous respiratory compromise, including smoking. **Multisystem failure** is not uncommon particularly in elderly patients with significant comorbidities. **Coagulopathy** is not uncommon when multisystem failure becomes established. **Lymphocele** or **lymph leakage** is not uncommon but is rarely a clinical problem. **Abdominal hernia formation** is not uncommon, sometimes developing years after surgery, and is associated with surgical wound infection. Embolism of debris to limbs or organs may cause irreversible ischemia causing **trash foot** and **limb or digit amputation** or **organ ischemia** and is another mechanism of organ failure (e.g., renal, cardiac, or gut complications). **Sexual dysfunction** may occur in both sexes but is less well documented in females.

Major Complications

The main serious complications of aortic aneurysm surgery result from bleeding, infection, or ischemia. Major **intraoperative** risks include serious **acute bleeding, cardiac failure,** and ischemia of limbs or organs, which can result in **circulatory collapse** when the aortic clamps are released at the procedure completion. Risk of **on-table death** is overall greater than for elective aortic repair procedures.

Postoperatively, there are considerable risks also mainly from **postoperative bleeding** and **hematoma formation**, sometimes resulting in **wound infection**. Rarely, **graft infection** may result in catastrophic **graft rupture** and **acute hemorrhage.** Graft infection may require graft removal and/or **re-operative bypass surgery.** Acute or chronic **graft thrombosis** may occur and can result in **ischemia, leg ulceration,** and even **limb/digit amputation. Loss of patency** can occur due to further disease at the anastomoses. **Severe leg edema** is a rare complication and may be assisted by stockings. **Sexual dysfunction** may occur due to inadvertent disruption of autonomic nerves; it may also predate surgery due to neurovascular disease. **Lymphoceles** are usually self-limited but sometimes require drainage and may predispose to infection. **Hernia formation** may occasionally result in **bowel obstruction** and require surgical repair. **Nerve injury** is rarely severe. **Aortoduodenal fistula** is a rare but catastrophic late complication, associated with acute melena, hematemesis, and/or severe hypotension. **Necrotizing fasciitis** is an extremely rare but devastating complication with a high mortality. **Renal failure** may require dialysis**, respiratory failure and ARDS** typically require prolonged ventilation, and **cardiac failure** may require inotropic and even pacemaker support. **Mesenteric ischemia** may require **bowel resection. GI bleeding, perforation, and stenosis of the bowel** may occur, requiring **further surgery. Multisystem organ failure** is a severe and often lethal complication related closely to preexisting pathology, comorbidities, and age.

Consent and Risk Reduction

Main Points to Explain

- Risks without surgery
- Pain
- Bleeding*
- Infection*
- Distal embolization*
- Organ failure
- ICU care
- Further surgery
- Death

*Dependent on pathology, graft, and site

Abdominal Aortic Aneurysm Repair:
Elective Endoluminal Aortic Stent Repair (EVAR)

Description

Local anesthetic and sedation, spinal, or general anesthesia is used. A percutaneous femoral approach via the groin or femoral artery cutdown is generally used. The aim is to enter the iliac vessels and abdominal aorta to permit placement of an endovascular stent inside the abdominal aortic aneurysm then expand the stent to create a new lumen within the aneurysm to restore flow with exclusion of the aneurysm sac to arterial blood flow. The graft is tested for seal and the catheter withdrawn.

Anatomical Points

The aortic and iliac anatomy may be highly distorted due to aneurysm formation, and branch points may be greatly disparate from the normal anatomical situation. The renal, mesenteric, gonadal, and iliac vessels may be rendered tortuous and asymmetrical, requiring careful identification. Lumbar vessels are variable in location and number and may cause type II endoleaks – "backfilling" the sac following stent graft placement. The graft is generally placed just below the renal arteries; however several currently available grafts have bare (open) stents at which sit above the renal arteries, allowing renal perfusion but improving device fixation. The sites of the spinal blood supply (arteries of Adamkiewicz; T1 and T11) are variable and occlusion may cause spinal ischemia and paralysis.

Perspective

See Table 3.11. Procedural success of endovascular AAA repair relies largely on the anatomical suitability of the aneurysm exclusion graft repair. The main

Table 3.11 Elective endoluminal aortic stent repair (EVAR): estimated frequency of complications, risks, and consequences

Complications, risks, and consequences	Estimated frequency
Most significant/serious complications	
Infection (overall)	2–5 %
Wound	1–5 %
Intra-abdominal	<2 %
Graft associated	1–5 %
Systemic sepsis	1–5 %

(continued)

Table 3.11 (continued)

Complications, risks, and consequences	Estimated frequency
Bleeding or hematoma formation[a]	
Wound	1–5 %
Graft associated	1–5 %
False aneurysm	1–5 %
Late graft failure tear dissection of artery, etc.	1–2 %
Graft thrombosis/blockage	1–5 %
Endoleak	
Type I	1–2 %
Type II	10–20 %
Type III	1–5 %
Type IV	1–2 %
Aneurysm rupture (per year)	0.3–1 %
Embolization	
Thrombus/atheroma	1–5 %
Paralysis and paraplegia	1–5 %
Cerebral ischemia/hemorrhage/thrombosis (CVA, TIA, RIND)[a]	1–5 %
Mesenteric ischemia	1–5 %
Colonic ischemia/necrosis[a]	1–5 %
Sexual dysfunction/impotence	5–20 %
Reactive thrombocythemia, leukocytosis	5–20 %
Small bowel obstruction (adhesions)	1–5 %
Renal impairment/failure	1–5 %
Myocardial impairment/failure[a]	1–5 %
Pulmonary impairment/failure	1–5 %
Multisystem failure (renal, pulmonary, cardiac failure)[a]	5–20 %
Death[a]	1–5 %
Rare significant/serious problems	
Neural injury	
Sensory (sciatic, ilioinguinal, femoral nerve/lat. cut. nerve thigh)	0.1–1 %
Motor (sciatic, femoral)	0.1–1 %
Erosion of arterial graft and major bleeding (late delayed bleeding)	0.1–1 %
Gut injury/perforation	0.1–1 %
Deep venous thrombosis/pulmonary embolus	0.1–1 %
Peripheral limb ischemia (trash foot/leg)[a]	0.1–1 %
Embolism to buttock muscle	0.1–1 %
Vascular injury[a]	
Femoral/iliac/renal/mesenteric artery or vein	0.1–1 %
Coagulopathy (DIC/consumption)	0.1–1 %
Abdominal compartment syndrome (may necessitate fasciotomy)	0.1–1 %
Limb compartment syndrome (may necessitate fasciotomy)	0.1–1 %
Paresthesia and/or muscle weakness	0.1–1 %
Femoral (or prevascular or inguinal) hernia (late aortoiliac or bifemoral aneurysm)	0.1–1 %
"Trash" kidney[a]	0.1–1 %
Cecal ulceration (aorto-bifemoral graft erosion)	<0.1 %
Gastrointestinal hemorrhage (aorto-enteric fistula or ischemic gut)	<0.1 %
Aorto-jejunal	<0.1 %
Aorto-cutaneous fistula[a]	<0.1 %

Table 3.11 (continued)

Complications, risks, and consequences	Estimated frequency
Aorto-caval fistula[a]	<0.1 %
Gas gangrene/necrotizing fasciitis[a]	<0.1 %
Less serious complications	
Skin ulceration	0.1–1 %
Chylous ascites/fistula	0.1–1 %
Orchitis/testicular atrophy[a]	0.1–1 %
Psychological changes[a] (often subtle)	5–20 %
Wound dehiscence	0.1–1 %
Paralytic ileus	50–80 %
Seroma/lymphatic fluid leak/lymphocele formation	1–5 %
Hyperbilirubinemia (unconjugated/thrombus related)	0.1–1 %
Leg edema swelling	1–5 %
Wound scarring/deformity – poor cosmesis	1–5 %
Blood transfusion[a]	1–5 %

[a]Dependent on underlying patient selection, pathology, anatomy, surgical technique, and preferences

complication of the procedure is endoleak (incomplete exclusion of the aneurysm sac from arterial blood flow). Endoleaks can be classified as type I (incomplete seal of graft proximally and distally) which requires urgent repair (endovascular or open) as the sac is at risk of rupture, type II endoleaks due to lumbar or inferior mesenteric vessels backfilling the sac (usually not treated), type III endoleaks (graft component disconnection), and type IV endoleak (graft porosity). Complications include bleeding, sometimes due to injury to the aorta or iliac vessels during stenting. Mesenteric ischemia due to inferior mesenteric artery occlusion may cause serious bowel complications, with or without the need for further surgery. Rarely, reperfusion injury due to restoration of arterial flow to the lower body may result in acidosis, release of products of ischemia, and hypotensive shock. Renal failure may be related to renal artery injury or coverage with graft or contrast-induced renal dysfunction can occur. Late thrombosis of the graft can cause distal ischemia and/or embolism. Respiratory infections are not uncommon, sometimes progressing to pneumonia and adult respiratory distress syndrome after prolonged surgery or previous respiratory compromise, including smoking. Multisystem organ failure is uncommon following EVAR. Coagulopathy is not uncommon when multisystem failure becomes established. Lymphocele or lymph leakage is not uncommon but is rarely a clinical problem. Embolism of debris to limbs may cause irreversible ischemia causing trash foot and limb or digit amputation or organ ischemia and is another mechanism or organ failure (e.g., renal, cardiac, or gut complications).

Major Complications

The main serious complications of aortic aneurysm surgery result from bleeding, infection, or ischemia. Major **intraoperative** risks include serious **acute bleeding, cardiac failure,** and **ischemia of limbs or organs**, which can result in **circulatory**

collapse when the aortic clamps are released at the procedure completion. Risk of **on-table death** (1–3 %) is overall less than for open aortic repair procedures.

Postoperatively, there are considerable risks also mainly from **postoperative bleeding** and **hematoma formation**, sometimes resulting in **wound infection**. Rarely, **graft infection** may result in catastrophic **graft rupture** and **acute hemorrhage.** Graft infection may require graft removal or **re-operative bypass surgery**. Acute or chronic **graft thrombosis** may occur and can result in **ischemia, leg ulceration,** and even **limb/digit amputation. Severe leg edema** is a rare complication and may be assisted by stockings. **Lymphoceles** are usually self-limited but sometimes require drainage and may predispose to infection. **Nerve injury** is rarely severe. **Aortoduodenal fistula** is a rare but catastrophic late complication associated with acute melena, hematemesis, and/or severe hypotension. **Necrotizing fasciitis** is an extremely rare but devastating complication with a high mortality. **Renal failure** may require dialysis**, respiratory failure and ARDS** typically require prolonged ventilation, and **cardiac failure** may require inotropic and even pacemaker support. **Mesenteric ischemia** may require **bowel resection. GI bleeding, perforation and stenosis of the bowel** may occur, requiring **further surgery. Multisystem organ failure** is a severe and often lethal complication related closely to preexisting comorbidities and age.

Consent and Risk Reduction

Main Points to Explain

- Pain
- Bleeding*
- Infection*
- Distal embolization*
- Graft failure
- Organ failure
- ICU care
- Further surgery
- Risks without surgery
- Death

*Dependent on pathology, graft, and site

Axillo-femoral Bypass Surgery

Description

General anesthetic is used. The aim is to bypass the obstructing lesion(s) in the aorta or common iliac artery. If femoral obstruction is present, a lower anastomosis may be possible. Axillo-femoral bypass graft is from the patent axillary artery to the patent ipsilateral femoral or iliac artery using synthetic graft material due to the length needed. Vertical incisions are generally made in the groin, with an oblique incision in the axilla, according to the site of obstruction and the relatively normal caliber vessels for anastomosis.

Anatomical Points

The axillary artery is typically uniform in its anatomy. The femoral and iliac arteries are relatively constant; however, the profunda femoris artery is moderately variable in location, especially in its origin. Angiography should usually map the divisions adequately. Pathology may cause stenosis, absence, and differing collateral circulation, which may alter anatomy significantly.

Perspective

See Table 3.12. Local wound problems, **hematoma, infection,** and **scarring,** are probably the most common complication of the axillo-femoral bypass graft surgery. The dual

Table 3.12 Axillo-femoral bypass graft surgery: estimated frequency of complications, risks, and consequences

Complications, risks, and consequences	Estimated frequency
Most significant/serious complications	
Bleeding or hematoma formation	
Wound(s)	1–5 %
Graft Dehiscence/leakage/rupture (early)[a] (including dissection of vessel wall; false aneurysm)	1–5 %
Late delayed bleeding (graft erosion)	0.1–1 %
Femoro-cutaneous fistula	<0.1 %
Early graft thrombosis/blockage[a]	1–5 %
Late graft failure (tearing, dissection, etc.)[a]	0.1–1 %
Embolization[a](thrombus or atheroma)	1–5 %
Limb amputation (short term)[a]	
Claudicants	1–5 %
Critical limb ischemia	5–20 %
Limb amputation (late)[a]	
Claudicants	5–20 %
Critical limb ischemia	20–50 %
Infection	
Wound[a]	5–20 %
Graft associated[a]	0.1–1 %
Systemic sepsis[a]	0.1–1 %
Wound dehiscence	1–5 %

(continued)

Table 3.12 (continued)

Complications, risks, and consequences	Estimated frequency
Seroma/lymphocele formation or lymphatic fluid leak	5–20 %
Myocardial impairment/infarction/failure[a]	1–5 %
Cerebral ischemia/hemorrhage/thrombosis (CVA, TIA, RIND)[a]	1–5 %
Neural injury[a] (overall)	1–5 %
Sensory (femoral nerve/lat. cut. nerve thigh/sciatic/axillary)	
Motor (femoral)	
Multisystem organ failure[a]	1–5 %
Death[a]	1–5 %
Rare significant/serious problems	
Limb compartment syndrome (may necessitate fasciotomy)[a]	<0.1 %
Vascular injury (femoral/axillary artery or vein)[a]	0.1–1 %
Peripheral limb ischemia (trash foot/leg)[a]	0.1–1 %
Deep venous thrombosis/pulmonary embolus	0.1–1 %
Gas gangrene/necrotizing fasciitis[a]	<0.1 %
Less serious complications	
Skin ulceration[a]	0.1–1 %
Femoral (or prevascular or inguinal) hernia (late)[a]	1–5 %
Leg/arm edema (long-term swelling)[a] (rarely severe)	5–20 %
Wound scarring/deformity – poor cosmesis	0.1–1 %
Blood transfusion[a]	0.1–1 %
Wound drainage tube[a]	1–5 %

[a]Dependent on underlying pathology, anatomy, surgical technique, comorbidities, and preferences

wound sites and long tunnelling procedure predisposes to increased risk of hematoma, infection, and wound complications. **Graft infection** is about 3 times greater for prosthetic (Dacron; PTFE) grafts than for autologous saphenous vein grafts. If graft infection occurs, occlusion rates, amputation rates, and mortality are significantly increased. **Nerve problems** are not uncommon and can cause chronic pain on occasions. Severe complications increase with time from surgery and include **thrombosis/embolism,** lower limb **distal ischemia re-operative bypass surgery,** and **amputation. Bleeding** risk is increased where thrombolytic agent infusions are used. **Lymphocele** or **lymph leakage** is not uncommon. **Graft occlusion**, **recurrent ischemia,** and **groin hernia formation**, often prevascular, are common later events with this surgery. Amputation risk increases in proportion to the extent of underlying distal vascular obstruction.

Major Complications

The major risks are **intraoperative** and **postoperative bleeding** and **hematoma formation, sometimes resulting in wound infection**. Rarely, graft infection may result in catastrophic **graft rupture** and **acute hemorrhage. Graft infection** may require graft removal. Acute or chronic **graft thrombosis** may occur and can result in **ischemia, ulceration, re-operative bypass surgery,** and **leg amputation. Loss of patency** typically occurs as time progresses, especially with long prosthetic grafts. **Amputation** risk increases as a function of vascular disease severity and time. **Severe leg or arm edema** is rarely severe and may be assisted by stockings and physiotherapy. **Lymphoceles** are usually self-limited but sometimes require repeated drainage and may predispose to infection. **Hernia formation** may occur if suprainguinal access is required and these are typically prevascular, occasionally resulting in **bowel obstruction**. **Further surgery** may be required for revascularization, amputation, hernia repair, or infection. **Nerve injury** is rarely severe, but both femoral and brachial sensory and motor nerve branches are at risk. **Necrotizing fasciitis** is an extremely rare but devastating complication with a high mortality.

Consent and Risk Reduction

Main Points to Explain

- Pain
- Bleeding*
- Infection*
- Distal embolization*
- Graft failure
- Organ failure
- ICU care
- Further surgery
- Risks without surgery
- Death

*Dependent on pathology, graft, and site

Thoracoscopic (Video-Assisted and Open) Sympathectomy

Description

Under general anesthesia with a double-lumen endobronchial tube in place, a small incision is made just beneath the axillary hairline (approximately the 3rd intercostal space) anterior to the midaxillary line. Via blunt dissection over the rib, the pleural space is entered once the ipsilateral lung is no longer ventilated. Video-assisted approaches are chiefly used, but occasionally open approaches are required. The aim is to divide the sympathetic chain usually over the 2nd rib but occasionally also over the 3rd and 4th ribs in the treatment of hyperhidrosis (most common indication and usually palmar), distal ischemia, or complex regional pain syndrome (reflex sympathetic dystrophy). Nerves of Kuntz are also divided when present. A chest X-ray is usually performed in the postoperative recovery room to detect any pneumothorax, which if significant may require a chest tube for drainage. The relative risks and complications of sympathectomy are primarily related to injury to the surrounding anatomy that lies close to the sympathetic chain. In general, thoracoscopic approaches have almost completely replaced open approaches because of the reduced morbidity with the minimal access procedures.

Anatomical Points

The intercostal neurovascular bundle lies inferior to each rib. Most sympathetic fibers supplying the upper limb emerge from the ventral roots of T2 or T3. The 1st rib is hidden by the apical fat pad and therefore the uppermost identifiable rib is the 2nd. The T2 ganglion lies between the 2nd and 3rd ribs. The sympathetic chain passes anterior to the necks of the ribs. The nerve of Kuntz contains sympathetic fibers travelling from the second intercostal nerve to the T1 nerve root, thus bypassing the T2 ganglion. These nerves occur in 10 % of the population and lie more laterally on the 2nd rib. The pleural cavity may be impeded by pleural adhesions, which may restrict access.

Perspective

See Table 3.13. The main serious complications are bleeding and infection, which can be minimized by the adequate exposure, mobilization, reduction of tension, and ensuring satisfactory blood supply to the distal tissues. Hemothorax and pneumothorax requiring intercostal drainage are uncommon. Massive hemothorax requiring thoracotomy occurs very infrequently. Infection is the main sequel of poor tissue perfusion or hematoma formation and may lead to abscess formation and systemic sepsis. Procedure failure is rare for palmar hyperhidrosis but more common in axillary hyperhidrosis. Sympathectomy is only rarely indicated for digital ischemia or complex regional pain syndromes, and in both conditions the results are very variable. Horner's syndrome may occur. Sympathetic compensatory sweating occurs more frequently in patients after bilateral than unilateral sympathectomy. Rare complications include chylous effusion, empyema, cardiac arrest, multisystem failure, and death (combined incidence 0.1–1 %). Postoperative pain may be severe, and rarely a neuroma of an intercostal nerve may develop causing chronic pain. Preexisting pleural adhesions may impede access and may increase the risk of lung injury, air leak, and postoperative pneumothorax.

Major Complications

Massive **hemothorax** requiring **thoracotomy**, although very rare, may result in **death**. **Horner's syndrome** (causing unequal pupils) is often very disturbing for the patient who has often sought treatment because of social anxiety. **Failure of the procedure** to alleviate hyperhidrosis or vascular spasm can be considered a major consequence of significance for the patient. **Basal atelectasis** and sometimes secondary **lung infection** is not uncommon and may affect either lung. Serious **lung infection** including **pneumonia** and **empyema** is uncommon but may be severe. **Lung injury** is rare, except where extensive pleural adhesions are present. **Cardiac**

Table 3.13 Thoracoscopic sympathectomy: estimated frequency of complications, risks, and consequences

Complications, risks, and consequences	Estimated frequency
Most significant/serious complications	
Infection	
Subcutaneous/wound	1–5 %
Intrathoracic (pneumonia; pleural)	1–5 %
Mediastinitis	<0.1 %
Systemic	<0.1 %
Pulmonary empyema	0.1–1 %
Bleeding and hematoma formation	
Wound	0.1–1 %
Hemothorax	0.1–1 %
Pulmonary contusion	0.1–1 %
Pneumothorax (residual)	1–5 %
Horner's syndrome[a]	1–5 %
Procedure failure	
For palmar hyperhidrosis	0.1–1 %
For axillary hyperhidrosis	5–20 %
Compensatory sweating (after unilateral sympathectomy)	20–50 %
Compensatory sweating (after bilateral sympathectomy)	50–80 %
Rare significant/serious problems	
Thoracotomy	0.1–1 %
Persistent air leak	0.1–1 %
Bronchopleural fistula	0.1–1 %
Cardiac arrhythmias	0.1–1 %
Pericardial effusion	0.1–1 %
Myocardial injury, cardiac failure, MI (hypotension)	0.1–1 %
Deep venous thrombosis	0.1–1 %
Diaphragmatic injury paresis (including phrenic nerve injury)[a]	< 0.1 %
Thoracic duct injury (chylous leak, fistula)	<0.1 %
Osteomyelitis of ribs[a]	<0.1 %
Pulmonary injury (direct or inferior pulmonary vein injury)	<0.1 %
Multisystem organ failure (renal, pulmonary, cardiac failure)[a]	0.1–1 %
Death	<0.1 %
Less serious complications	
Surgical emphysema	0.1–1 %
Rib pain, wound pain	
Acute (<4 weeks)	50–80 %
Chronic (>12 weeks)	0.1–1 %
Neuroma formation[a]	0.1–1 %
Wound scarring or port site or minithoracotomy	1–5 %
Deformity of rib or skin (poor cosmesis)	1–5 %
Pleural drain tube(s)[a]	5–20 %

[a]Dependent on underlying anatomy, pathology, location of disease, and/or surgical preference

events, including arrhythmias, myocardial infarction, and cardiac arrest can occur and may rarely be lethal. However, **multisystem organ failure** is exceedingly rare as is **death** from this or any cause. **Neural injuries** (other than the desired division of the sympathetic chain) are potential associated problems with this surgery as is **vascular injury**, because vessels are commonly anatomically close to nerves and are at risk of injury during dissection.

Consent and Risk Reduction

Main Points to Explain

- Discomfort
- Bleeding
- Procedure failure
- Horner's syndrome
- Compensatory sweating
- Lung infection
- Further surgery
- Risks without surgery

Further Reading, References, and Resources

Diagnostic Angiography

Barrett BJ. Contrast-induced nephropathy: we need all the data to discern the truth. Am J Kidney Dis. 2009;54(4):587–9.

Clemente CD. Anatomy – a regional atlas of the human body. 4th ed. Baltimore: Williams and Wilkins; 1997.

Jamieson GG. The anatomy of general surgical operations. 2nd ed. Edinburgh: Churchill Livingston; 2006.

Patel ST, Mills Sr JL, Tynan-Cuisinier G, Goshima KR, Westerband A, Westerband A, Hughes JD. The limitations of magnetic resonance angiography in the diagnosis of renal artery stenosis: comparative analysis with conventional arteriography. J Vasc Surg. 2005;41(3):462–8.

Peck MA, Conrad MF, Kwolek CJ, Lamuraglia GM, Paruchuri V, Cambria RP. Intermediate-term outcomes of endovascular treatment for symptomatic chronic mesenteric ischemia. J Vasc Surg. 2010;51(1):140–7. e1-2.

Thiex R, Norbash AM, Frerichs KU. The safety of dedicated-team catheter-based diagnostic cerebral angiography in the era of advanced noninvasive imaging. AJNR Am J Neuroradiol. 2010;31(2):230–4.

Temporal Artery Biopsy

Clemente CD. Anatomy – a regional atlas of the human body. 4th ed. Baltimore: Williams and Wilkins; 1997.

Jamieson GG. The anatomy of general surgical operations. 2nd ed. Edinburgh: Churchill Livingston; 2006.

Arteriovenous Fistula Surgery

Clemente CD. Anatomy – a regional atlas of the human body. 4th ed. Baltimore: Williams and Wilkins; 1997.

Conlon PJ, Schwab SJ, Nicholson ML, editors. Hemodialysis vascular access: practice and problems. Oxford: Oxford University Press; 2000.

Jamieson GG. The anatomy of general surgical operations. 2nd ed. Edinburgh: Churchill Livingston; 2006.

Lauvao LS, Ihnat DM, Goshima KR, Chavez L, Gruessner AC, Mills Sr JL. Vein diameter is the major predictor of fistula maturation. J Vasc Surg. 2009;49(6):1499–504.

Levy J., Morgan J. Brown E, editors. Haemodialysis – Chapter in Oxford handbook of dialysis. Oxford: Oxford University Press; 2001.

Murphy GJ, White SA, Nicholson ML. Vascular access for haemodialysis. Br J Surg. 2000;87: 1300–15.

Nicholson ML., White S. Access for renal replacement therapy. In: Morris PJ, editor. Kidney transplantation: principles and practices. 5th ed. Philadelphia: WB Saunders; 2001.

Brachial Embolectomy (Including Graft Embolectomy)

Clemente CD. Anatomy – a regional atlas of the human body. 4th ed. Baltimore: Williams and Wilkins; 1997.

Jamieson GG. The anatomy of general surgical operations. 2nd ed. Edinburgh: Churchill Livingston; 2006.

Femoropopliteal Embolectomy (Including Graft Embolectomy)

Clemente CD. Anatomy – a regional atlas of the human body. 4th ed. Baltimore: Williams and Wilkins; 1997.

Jamieson GG. The anatomy of general surgical operations. 2nd ed. Edinburgh: Churchill Livingston; 2006.

Mesenteric Arterial Embolectomy

Clemente CD. Anatomy – a regional atlas of the human body. 4th ed. Baltimore: Williams and Wilkins; 1997.

Jamieson GG. The anatomy of general surgical operations. 2nd ed. Edinburgh: Churchill Livingston; 2006.

Peck MA, Conrad MF, Kwolek CJ, Lamuraglia GM, Paruchuri V, Cambria RP. Intermediate-term outcomes of endovascular treatment for symptomatic chronic mesenteric ischemia. J Vasc Surg. 2010;51(1):140–7. e1-2.

Schermerhorn ML, Giles KA, Hamdan AD, Wyers MC, Pomposelli FB. Mesenteric revascularization: management and outcomes in the United States, 1988–2006. J Vasc Surg. 2009;50(2): 341–8. e1.

Carotid Endarterectomy

Ahmed B, Al-Khaffaf H. Prevalence of significant asymptomatic carotid artery disease in patients with peripheral vascular disease: a meta-analysis. Eur J Vasc Endovasc Surg. 2009; 37(3):262–71. Review.

Beckett D, Gaines PA. Lessons from EVA-3S and SPACE. Cardiovasc Intervent Radiol. 2008;31(1):5–7. Review.

Brahmanandam S, Ding EL, Conte MS, Belkin M, Nguyen LL. Clinical results of carotid artery stenting compared with carotid endarterectomy. J Vasc Surg. 2008;47(2):343–9. Review.

Clemente CD. Anatomy – a regional atlas of the human body. 4th ed. Baltimore: Williams and Wilkins; 1997.

Ederle J, Featherstone RL, Brown MM. Percutaneous transluminal angioplasty and stenting for carotid artery stenosis. Cochrane Database Syst Rev. 2007;(4):CD000515. Review.

Ederle J, Featherstone RL, Brown MM. Randomized controlled trials comparing endarterectomy and endovascular treatment for carotid artery stenosis: a Cochrane systematic review. Stroke. 2009;40(4):1373–80. Review.

Gurm HS, Nallamothu BK, Yadav J. Safety of carotid artery stenting for symptomatic carotid artery disease: a meta-analysis. Eur Heart J. 2008;29(1):113–9. Review.

Holt PJ, Poloniecki JD, Loftus IM, Thompson MM. Meta-analysis and systematic review of the relationship between hospital volume and outcome following carotid endarterectomy. Eur J Vasc Endovasc Surg. 2007;33(6):645–51. Review.

Jamieson GG. The anatomy of general surgical operations. 2nd ed. Edinburgh: Churchill Livingston; 2006.

Jeng JS, Liu HM, Tu YK. Carotid angioplasty with or without stenting versus carotid endarterectomy for carotid artery stenosis: a meta-analysis. J Neurol Sci. 2008;270(1–2):40–7.

Killeen SD, Andrews EJ, Redmond HP, Fulton GJ. Provider volume and outcomes for abdominal aortic aneurysm repair, carotid endarterectomy, and lower extremity revascularization procedures. J Vasc Surg. 2007;45(3):615–26. Review.

Lip GY, Kalra L. Stroke prevention. Clin Evid (Online). 2008;2008:pii: 0207.

Mortaz Hejri S, Mostafazadeh Davani B, Sahraian MA. Carotid endarterectomy for carotid stenosis in patients selected for coronary artery bypass graft surgery. Cochrane Database Syst Rev. 2009;(4):CD006074.

Murad MH, Flynn DN, Elamin MB, Guyatt GH, Hobson 2nd RW, Erwin PJ, Montori VM. Endarterectomy vs stenting for carotid artery stenosis: a systematic review and meta-analysis. J Vasc Surg. 2008;48(2):487–93. Review.

Naylor AR. ICSS and EXACT/CAPTURE: more questions than answers. Eur J Vasc Endovasc Surg. 2009;38(4):397–401.

Rerkasem K, Rothwell PM. Local versus general anaesthesia for carotid endarterectomy. Cochrane Database Syst Rev. 2008;(4):CD000126. Review.

Rerkasem K, Rothwell PM. Patch angioplasty versus primary closure for carotid endarterectomy. Cochrane Database Syst Rev. 2009;(4):CD000160.

Rerkasem K, Rothwell PM. Routine or selective carotid artery shunting for carotid endarterectomy (and different methods of monitoring in selective shunting). Cochrane Database Syst Rev. 2009;(4):CD000190.

Seretis K, Goudakos I, Vlachakis I, Anthimidis G, Papadimitriou D. Carotid artery disease in octogenarians: endarterectomy or stenting? Int Angiol. 2007;26(4):353–60. Review.

Timaran CH, Rosero EB, Smith ST, Valentine RJ, Modrall JG, Clagett GP. Trends and outcomes of concurrent carotid revascularization and coronary bypass. J Vasc Surg. 2008;48(2):355–60. discussion 360–1.

van der Vaart MG, Meerwaldt R, Reijnen MM, Tio RA, Zeebregts CJ. Endarterectomy or carotid artery stenting: the quest continues. Am J Surg. 2008;195(2):259–69. Review.

Wolff T, Guirguis-Blake J, Miller T, Gillespie M, Harris R. Screening for carotid artery stenosis: an update of the evidence for the U.S. Preventive Services Task Force. Ann Intern Med. 2007;147(12):860–70. Review.

Wong EH, Farrier JN, Cooper DG. First-bite syndrome complicating carotid endarterectomy: a case report and literature review. Vasc Endovasc Surg. 2011;45(5):459–61.

Femoropopliteal Bypass Surgery

Aulivola B, Pomposelli FB. Dorsalis pedis, tarsal and plantar artery bypass. J Cardiovasc Surg (Torino). 2004;45(3):203–12. Review.

Clemente CD. Anatomy – a regional atlas of the human body. 4th ed. Baltimore: Williams and Wilkins; 1997.

Domenig CM, Hamdan AD, Holzenbein TJ, Kansal N, Aulivola B, Skillman JJ, Campbell DR, LoGerfo FW, Pomposelli Jr FB. Timing of pedal bypass failure and its impact on the need for amputation. Ann Vasc Surg. 2005;19(1):56–62.

Giles KA, Hamdan AD, Pomposelli FB, Wyers MC, Siracuse JJ, Schermerhorn ML. Body mass index: surgical site infections and mortality after lower extremity bypass from the National Surgical Quality Improvement Program 2005–2007. Ann Vasc Surg. 2010;24(1): 48–56.

Goshima KR, Mills Sr JL, Hughes JD. A new look at outcomes after infrainguinal bypass surgery: traditional reporting standards systematically underestimate the expenditure of effort required to attain limb salvage. J Vasc Surg. 2004;39(2):330–5.

Herrera FA, Kohanzadeh S, Nasseri Y, Kansal N, Owens EL, Bodor R. Management of vascular graft infections with soft tissue flap coverage: improving limb salvage rates–a veterans affairs experience. Am Surg. 2009;75(10):877–81.

Ihnat DM, Duong ST, Taylor ZC, Leon LR, Mills Sr JL, Goshima KR, Echeverri JA, Arslan B. Contemporary outcomes after superficial femoral artery angioplasty and stenting: the influence of TASC classification and runoff score. J Vasc Surg. 2008;47(5):967–74.

Jackson MJ, Wolfe JH. Are infra-inguinal angioplasty and surgery comparable? Acta Chir Belg. 2001;101(1):6–10. Review.

Jamieson GG. The anatomy of general surgical operations. 2nd ed. Edinburgh: Churchill Livingston; 2006.

Killeen SD, Andrews EJ, Redmond HP, Fulton GJ. Provider volume and outcomes for abdominal aortic aneurysm repair, carotid endarterectomy, and lower extremity revascularization procedures. J Vasc Surg. 2007;45(3):615–26. Review.

Klinkert P, Post PN, Breslau PJ, van Bockel JH. Saphenous vein versus PTFE for above-knee femoropopliteal bypass. A review of the literature. Eur J Vasc Endovasc Surg. 2004;27(4): 357–62. Review.

Lumsden AB, Davies MG, Peden EK. Medical and endovascular management of critical limb ischemia. J Endovasc Ther. 2009;16(2 Suppl 2):II31–62. Review.

Met R, Van Lienden KP, Koelemay MJ, Bipat S, Legemate DA, Reekers JA. Subintimal angioplasty for peripheral arterial occlusive disease: a systematic review. Cardiovasc Intervent Radiol. 2008;31(4):687–97. Review.

Perera GB, Lyden SP. Current trends in lower extremity revascularization. Surg Clin North Am. 2007;87(5):1135–47. x. Review.

Pomposelli FB, Kansal N, Hamdan AD, Belfield A, Sheahan M, Campbell DR, Skillman JJ, Logerfo FW. A decade of experience with dorsalis pedis artery bypass: analysis of outcome in more than 1000 cases. J Vasc Surg. 2003;37(2):307–15.

Ramdev P, Rayan SS, Sheahan M, Hamdan AD, Logerfo FW, Akbari CM, Campbell DR, Pomposelli Jr FB. A decade experience with infrainguinal revascularization in a dialysis-dependent patient population. J Vasc Surg. 2002;36(5):969–74.

Sheahan MG, Hamdan AD, Veraldi JR, McArthur CS, Skillman JJ, Campbell DR, Scovell SD, Logerfo FW, Pomposelli Jr FB. Lower extremity minor amputations: the roles of diabetes mellitus and timing of revascularization. J Vasc Surg. 2005;42(3):476–80.

Silver MJ, Ansel GM. Femoropopliteal occlusive disease: diagnosis, indications for treatment, and results of interventional therapy. Catheter Cardiovasc Interv. 2002;56(4):555–61. Review.

Simosa HF, Pomposelli FB, Dahlberg S, Scali ST, Hamdan AD, Schermerhorn ML. Predictors of failure after angioplasty of infrainguinal vein bypass grafts. J Vasc Surg. 2009a;49(1): 117–21.

Simosa HF, Malek JY, Schermerhorn ML, Giles KA, Pomposelli FB, Hamdan AD. Endoluminal intervention for limb salvage after failed lower extremity bypass graft. J Vasc Surg. 2009b; 49(6):1426–30.

Elective Abdominal Aortic/Iliac Aneurysm Repair

Ballard DJ, Filardo G, Fowkes G, Powell JT. Surgery for small asymptomatic abdominal aortic aneurysms. Cochrane Database Syst Rev. 2008;(4):CD001835. Review.

Brooke BS, Perler BA, Dominici F, Makary MA, Pronovost PJ. Reduction of in-hospital mortality among California hospitals meeting Leapfrog evidence-based standards for abdominal aortic aneurysm repair. J Vasc Surg. 2008;47(6):1155–6. discussion 1163–4.

Clemente CD. Anatomy – a regional atlas of the human body. 4th ed. Baltimore: Williams and Wilkins; 1997.

Cosford PA, Leng GC. Screening for abdominal aortic aneurysm. Cochrane Database Syst Rev. 2007;(2):CD002945. Review.

Dillavou ED, Muluk SC, Makaroun MS. A decade of change in abdominal aortic aneurysm repair in the United States: have we improved outcomes equally between men and women? J Vasc Surg. 2006;43(2):230–8. discussion 238.

Ehlers L, Sørensen J, Jensen LG, Bech M, Kjølby M. Is population screening for abdominal aortic aneurysm cost-effective? BMC Cardiovasc Disord. 2008;8:32.

Ehlers L, Overvad K, Sørensen J, Christensen S, Bech M, Kjølby M. Analysis of cost effectiveness of screening Danish men aged 65 for abdominal aortic aneurysm. BMJ. 2009;338:b2243. doi:10.1136/bmj.b2243.

Goshima KR, Mills Sr JL, Awari K, Pike SL, Hughes JD. Measure what matters: institutional outcome data are superior to the use of surrogate markers to define "center of excellence" for abdominal aortic aneurysm repair. Ann Vasc Surg. 2008;22(3):328–34.

Grant MW, Thomson IA, van Rij AM. In-hospital mortality of ruptured abdominal aortic aneurysm. ANZ J Surg. 2008;78(8):698–704.

Hagihara PF, Ernst CB, Griffen Jr WO. Incidence of ischemic colitis following abdominal aortic reconstruction. Surg Gynecol Obstet. 1979;149(4):571–3.

Henebiens M, van den Broek TA, Vahl AC, Koelemay MJ. Relation between hospital volume and outcome of elective surgery for abdominal aortic aneurysm: a systematic review. Eur J Vasc Endovasc Surg. 2007;33(3):285–92. Review.

Henebiens M, Vahl A, Koelemay MJ. Elective surgery of abdominal aortic aneurysms in octogenarians: a systematic review. J Vasc Surg. 2008;47(3):676–81.

Hertzer NR, Beven EG, Young JR, O'Hara PJ, Ruschhaupt 3rd WF, Graor RA, et al. Coronary artery disease in peripheral vascular patients. A classification of 1000 coronary angiograms and results of surgical management. Ann Surg. 1984;199(2):223–33.

Hertzer NR, Young JR, Beven EG, O'Hara PJ, Graor RA, Ruschhaupt WF, et al. Late results of coronary bypass in patients with infrarenal aortic aneurysms. The Cleveland Clinic Study. Ann Surg. 1987;205(4):360–7.

Holt PJ, Poloniecki JD, Loftus IM, Thompson MM. Meta-analysis and systematic review of the relationship between hospital volume and outcome following carotid endarterectomy. Eur J Vasc Endovasc Surg. 2007;33(6):645–51. Review.

Hopkins R, Bowen J, Campbell K, Blackhouse G, De Rose G, Novick T, et al. Effects of study design and trends for EVAR versus OSR. Vasc Health Risk Manag. 2008;4(5):1011–22. Review.

Jamieson GG. The anatomy of general surgical operations. 2nd ed. Edinburgh: Churchill Livingston; 2006.

Jonker FH, Schlösser FJ, Moll FL, Muhs BE. Dissection of the abdominal aorta. Current evidence and implications for treatment strategies: a review and meta-analysis of 92 patients. J Endovasc Ther. 2009;16(1):71–80. Review.

Kazmers A, Jacobs L, Perkins A, Lindenauer SM, Bates E. Abdominal aortic aneurysm repair in Veterans Affairs medical centers. J Vasc Surg. 1996;23(2):191–200.

Killeen SD, Andrews EJ, Redmond HP, Fulton GJ. Provider volume and outcomes for abdominal aortic aneurysm repair, carotid endarterectomy, and lower extremity revascularization procedures. J Vasc Surg. 2007;45(3):615–26. Review.

Lederle FA, Kane RL, MacDonald R, Wilt TJ. Systematic review: repair of unruptured abdominal aortic aneurysm. Ann Intern Med. 2007;146(10):735–41. Review.

Lederle FA, Larson JC, Margolis KL, Allison MA, Freiberg MS, Cochrane BB, et al. Abdominal aortic aneurysm events in the women's health initiative: cohort study. BMJ. 2008;337:a1724. doi:10.1136/bmj.a1724.

Mills Sr JL, Duong ST, Leon Jr LR, Goshima KR, Ihnat DM, Wendel CS, Gruessner A. Comparison of the effects of open and endovascular aortic aneurysm repair on long-term renal function using chronic kidney disease staging based on glomerular filtration rate. J Vasc Surg. 2008;47(6):1141–9.

Patterson BO, Holt PJ, Hinchliffe R, Loftus IM, Thompson MM. Predicting risk in elective abdominal aortic aneurysm repair: a systematic review of current evidence. Eur J Vasc Endovasc Surg. 2008;36(6):637–45. Review.

Rigberg DA, Zingmond DS, McGory ML, Maggard MA, Agustin M, Lawrence PF, et al. Age stratified, perioperative, and one-year mortality after abdominal aortic aneurysm repair: a statewide experience. J Vasc Surg. 2006;43(2):224–9

Tambyraja AL, Murie JA, Chalmers RT. Prediction of outcome after abdominal aortic aneurysm rupture. J Vasc Surg. 2008;47(1):222–30. Review.

van Prehn J, Schlösser FJ, Muhs BE, Verhagen HJ, Moll FL, van Herwaarden JA. Oversizing of aortic stent grafts for abdominal aneurysm repair: a systematic review of the benefits and risks. Eur J Vasc Endovasc Surg. 2009;38(1):42–53. Review.

Wilt TJ, Lederle FA, Macdonald R, Jonk YC, Rector TS, Kane RL. Comparison of endovascular and open surgical repairs for abdominal aortic aneurysm. Evid Rep Technol Assess (Full Rep). 2006;144:1–113. Review.

Young EL, Holt PJ, Poloniecki JD, Loftus IM, Thompson MM. Meta-analysis and systematic review of the relationship between surgeon annual caseload and mortality for elective open abdominal aortic aneurysm repairs. J Vasc Surg. 2007;46(6):1287–94. Review.

Emergency Abdominal Aortic/Iliac Aneurysm Repair

Ballard DJ, Filardo G, Fowkes G, Powell JT. Surgery for small asymptomatic abdominal aortic aneurysms. Cochrane Database Syst Rev. 2008;(4):CD001835. Review.

Brooke BS, Perler BA, Dominici F, Makary MA, Pronovost PJ. Reduction of in-hospital mortality among California hospitals meeting Leapfrog evidence-based standards for abdominal aortic aneurysm repair. J Vasc Surg. 2008;47(6):1155–6. discussion 1163–4.

Clemente CD. Anatomy – a regional atlas of the human body. 4th ed. Baltimore: Williams and Wilkins; 1997.

Cosford PA, Leng GC. Screening for abdominal aortic aneurysm. Cochrane Database Syst Rev. 2007;(2):CD002945. Review.

Dillavou ED, Muluk SC, Makaroun MS. A decade of change in abdominal aortic aneurysm repair in the United States: have we improved outcomes equally between men and women? J Vasc Surg. 2006;43(2):230–8. discussion 238.

Ehlers L, Sørensen J, Jensen LG, Bech M, Kjølby M. Is population screening for abdominal aortic aneurysm cost-effective? BMC Cardiovasc Disord. 2008;8:32.

Ehlers L, Overvad K, Sørensen J, Christensen S, Bech M, Kjølby M. Analysis of cost effectiveness of screening Danish men aged 65 for abdominal aortic aneurysm. BMJ. 2009;338:b2243. doi:10.1136/bmj.b2243.

Goshima KR, Mills Sr JL, Awari K, Pike SL, Hughes JD. Measure what matters: institutional outcome data are superior to the use of surrogate markers to define "center of excellence" for abdominal aortic aneurysm repair. Ann Vasc Surg. 2008;22(3):328–34.

Grant MW, Thomson IA, van Rij AM. In-hospital mortality of ruptured abdominal aortic aneurysm. ANZ J Surg. 2008;78(8):698–704.

Hagihara PF, Ernst CB, Griffen Jr WO. Incidence of ischemic colitis following abdominal aortic reconstruction. Surg Gynecol Obstet. 1979;149(4):571–3.

Henebiens M, van den Broek TA, Vahl AC, Koelemay MJ. Relation between hospital volume and outcome of elective surgery for abdominal aortic aneurysm: a systematic review. Eur J Vasc Endovasc Surg. 2007;33(3):285–92. Review.

Henebiens M, Vahl A, Koelemay MJ. Elective surgery of abdominal aortic aneurysms in octogenarians: a systematic review. J Vasc Surg. 2008;47(3):676–81.

Hertzer NR, Beven EG, Young JR, O'Hara PJ, Ruschhaupt 3rd WF, Graor RA, et al. Coronary artery disease in peripheral vascular patients. A classification of 1000 coronary angiograms and results of surgical management. Ann Surg. 1984;199(2):223–33.

Hertzer NR, Young JR, Beven EG, O'Hara PJ, Graor RA, Ruschhaupt WF, et al. Late results of coronary bypass in patients with infrarenal aortic aneurysms. The Cleveland Clinic Study. Ann Surg. 1987;205(4):360–7.

Holt PJ, Poloniecki JD, Loftus IM, Thompson MM. Meta-analysis and systematic review of the relationship between hospital volume and outcome following carotid endarterectomy. Eur J Vasc Endovasc Surg. 2007;33(6):645–51. Review.

Hopkins R, Bowen J, Campbell K, Blackhouse G, De Rose G, Novick T, et al. Effects of study design and trends for EVAR versus OSR. Vasc Health Risk Manag. 2008;4(5):1011–22. Review.

Jamieson GG. The anatomy of general surgical operations. 2nd ed. Edinburgh: Churchill Livingston; 2006.

Jonker FH, Schlösser FJ, Moll FL, Muhs BE. Dissection of the abdominal aorta. Current evidence and implications for treatment strategies: a review and meta-analysis of 92 patients. J Endovasc Ther. 2009;16(1):71–80. Review.

Kazmers A, Jacobs L, Perkins A, Lindenauer SM, Bates E. Abdominal aortic aneurysm repair in Veterans Affairs medical centers. J Vasc Surg. 1996;23(2):191–200.

Killeen SD, Andrews EJ, Redmond HP, Fulton GJ. Provider volume and outcomes for abdominal aortic aneurysm repair, carotid endarterectomy, and lower extremity revascularization procedures. J Vasc Surg. 2007;45(3):615–26. Review.

Lederle FA, Kane RL, MacDonald R, Wilt TJ. Systematic review: repair of unruptured abdominal aortic aneurysm. Ann Intern Med. 2007;146(10):735–41. Review.

Lederle FA, Larson JC, Margolis KL, Allison MA, Freiberg MS, Cochrane BB, et al. Abdominal aortic aneurysm events in the women's health initiative: cohort study. BMJ. 2008;337:a1724. doi:10.1136/bmj.a1724.

Patterson BO, Holt PJ, Hinchliffe R, Loftus IM, Thompson MM. Predicting risk in elective abdominal aortic aneurysm repair: a systematic review of current evidence. Eur J Vasc Endovasc Surg. 2008;36(6):637–45. Review.

Rigberg DA, Zingmond DS, McGory ML, Maggard MA, Agustin M, Lawrence PF, et al. Age stratified, perioperative, and one-year mortality after abdominal aortic aneurysm repair: a statewide experience. J Vasc Surg. 2006;43(2):224–9

Tambyraja AL, Murie JA, Chalmers RT. Prediction of outcome after abdominal aortic aneurysm rupture. J Vasc Surg. 2008;47(1):222–30. Review.

van Prehn J, Schlösser FJ, Muhs BE, Verhagen HJ, Moll FL, van Herwaarden JA. Oversizing of aortic stent grafts for abdominal aneurysm repair: a systematic review of the benefits and risks. Eur J Vasc Endovasc Surg. 2009;38(1):42–53. Review.

Wilt TJ, Lederle FA, Macdonald R, Jonk YC, Rector TS, Kane RL. Comparison of endovascular and open surgical repairs for abdominal aortic aneurysm. Evid Rep Technol Assess (Full Rep). 2006;144:1–113. Review.

Young EL, Holt PJ, Poloniecki JD, Loftus IM, Thompson MM. Meta-analysis and systematic review of the relationship between surgeon annual caseload and mortality for elective open abdominal aortic aneurysm repairs. J Vasc Surg. 2007;46(6):1287–94. Review.

Elective Endoluminal Aortic Stent Repair (EVAR)

Chahwan S, Comerota AJ, Pigott JP, Scheuermann BW, Burrow J, Wojnarowski D. Elective treatment of abdominal aortic aneurysm with endovascular or open repair: the first decade. J Vasc Surg. 2007;45(2):258–62. discussion 262.

Clemente CD. Anatomy – a regional atlas of the human body. 4th ed. Baltimore: Williams and Wilkins; 1997.

Davis M, Taylor PR. Endovascular infrarenal abdominal aortic aneurysm repair. Heart. 2008;94(2):222–8. Review.

Henebiens M, van den Broek TA, Vahl AC, Koelemay MJ. Relation between hospital volume and outcome of elective surgery for abdominal aortic aneurysm: a systematic review. Eur J Vasc Endovasc Surg. 2007;33(3):285–92. Review.

Hopkins R, Bowen J, Campbell K, Blackhouse G, De Rose G, Novick T, et al. Effects of study design and trends for EVAR versus OSR. Vasc Health Risk Manag. 2008;4(5):1011–22. Review.

Jamieson GG. The anatomy of general surgical operations. 2nd ed. Edinburgh: Churchill Livingston; 2006.

Jonker FH, Schlösser FJ, Moll FL, Muhs BE. Dissection of the abdominal aorta. Current evidence and implications for treatment strategies: a review and meta-analysis of 92 patients. J Endovasc Ther. 2009;16(1):71–80. Review.

Lederle FA, Kane RL, MacDonald R, Wilt TJ. Systematic review: repair of unruptured abdominal aortic aneurysm. Ann Intern Med. 2007;146(10):735–41. Review.

Monge M, Eskandari MK. Strategies for ruptured abdominal aortic aneurysms. J Vasc Interv Radiol. 2008;19(6 Suppl):S44–50.

Paolini D, Chahwan S, Wojnarowski D, Pigott JP, LaPorte F, Comerota AJ. Elective endovascular and open repair of abdominal aortic aneurysms in octogenarians. J Vasc Surg. 2008;47(5):924–7.

Prusa AM, Wolff KS, Sahal M, Polterauer P, Lammer J, Kretschmer G, Huk I, Teufelsbauer H. Abdominal aortic aneurysms and concomitant diseases requiring surgical intervention: simultaneous operation vs staged treatment using endoluminal stent grafting. Arch Surg. 2005;140(7):686–91.

Sheehan MK, Marone L, Makaroun MS. Use of endoluminal aortic stent-grafts for the repair of abdominal aortic aneurysms. Perspect Vasc Surg Endovasc Ther. 2005;17(4):289–96. Review.

van Prehn J, Schlösser FJ, Muhs BE, Verhagen HJ, Moll FL, van Herwaarden JA. Oversizing of aortic stent grafts for abdominal aneurysm repair: a systematic review of the benefits and risks. Eur J Vasc Endovasc Surg. 2009;38(1):42–53. Review.

Wilt TJ, Lederle FA, Macdonald R, Jonk YC, Rector TS, Kane RL. Comparison of endovascular and open surgical repairs for abdominal aortic aneurysm. Evid Rep Technol Assess (Full Rep). 2006;144:1–113. Review.

Axillo-femoral Bypass Graft Surgery

Arvanitis DP, Georgopoulos SE, Dervisis KI, Xanthopoulos DK, Lazarides MK. Early disruption of proximal anastomosis of a PTFE axillofemoral bypass graft. Vasa. 2002;31(2):136–7.

Chen IM, Chang HH, Hsu CP, Lai ST, Shih CC. Ten-year experience with surgical repair of mycotic aortic aneurysms. J Chin Med Assoc. 2005;68(6):265–71.

Clemente CD. Anatomy – a regional atlas of the human body. 4th ed. Baltimore: Williams and Wilkins; 1997.

Jamieson GG. The anatomy of general surgical operations. 2nd ed. Edinburgh: Churchill Livingston; 2006.

Järvinen A, Ketonen P, Meurala H, Harjola PT. Lower extremity revascularisation with axillo-femoral bypass grafting in 28 patients. Ann Chir Gynaecol. 1980;69(2):54–9.

Johnson WC, Squires JW. Axillo-femoral (PTFE) and infrainguinal revascularization (PTFE and umbilical vein). Vascular Registry of the New England Society for Vascular Surgery. J Cardiovasc Surg (Torino). 1991;32(3):344–9.

Kanemitsu S, Shimono T, Onoda K, Shimpo H. Temporary axillo-femoral bypass for abdominal aortic aneurysm repair in high risk patients. Ann Thorac Cardiovasc Surg. 2006;12(1):71–3.

Laohapensang K, Pongcheowboon A. A simple tunneler for extra-anatomical bypass grafts and interposition arteriovenous hemodialysis fistulas. J Med Assoc Thai. 1994;77(4):195–200.

Livesay JJ, Atkinson JB, Baker JD, Busuttil RW, Barker WF, Machleder HI. Late results of extra-anatomic bypass. Arch Surg. 1979;114(11):1260–7.

Madiba TE, Abdool-Carrim AT, Mars M, Nair R, Robbs JV. Management of graft occlusion following aortobifemoral bypass. Cardiovasc J S Afr. 2000;11(2):77–80.

Olah A, Vogt M, Laske A, Carrell T, Bauer E, Turina M. Axillo-femoral bypass and simultaneous removal of the aorto-femoral vascular infection site: is the procedure safe? Eur J Vasc Surg. 1992;6(3):252–4.

Rashleigh-Belcher HJ, Newcombe JF. Axillary artery thrombosis: a complication of axillo-femoral bypass grafts. Surgery. 1987;101(3):373–5.

Stain SC, Weaver FA, Yellin AE. Extra-anatomic bypass of failed traumatic arterial repairs. J Trauma. 1991;31(4):575–8.

Vijayanagar R, Bognolo DA, Eckstein PF. Extra-anatomic bypass operation for aorto-iliac disease in poor risk cardio-pulmonary patients. Angiology. 1982;33(11):695–701.

Thoracic Sympathectomy

Allen AY, Meyer DR. Neck procedures resulting in Horner syndrome. Ophthal Plast Reconstr Surg. 2009;25(1):16–8.

Backman SB. Regional anesthesia: sympathectomy-mediated vasodilation. Can J Anaesth. 2009;56(9):702–3. author reply 703.

Bachmann K, Standl N, Kaifi J, Busch P, Winkler E, Mann O, Izbicki JR, Strate T. Thoracoscopic sympathectomy for palmar and axillary hyperhidrosis: four-year outcome and quality of life after bilateral 5-mm dual port approach. Surg Endosc. 2009;23(7):1587–93.

Bakst R, Merola JF, Franks Jr AG, Sanchez M. Raynaud's phenomenon: pathogenesis and management. J Am Acad Dermatol. 2008;59(4):633–53. Review.

Baue AE. Glen's thoracic & cardiovascular surgery. 6th ed. Connecticut: Appleton & Lange; 1996.

Chen YB, Ye W, Yang WT, Shi L, Guo XF, Xu ZH, Qian YY. Uniportal versus biportal video-assisted thoracoscopic sympathectomy for palmar hyperhidrosis. Chin Med J (Engl). 2009;122(13):1525–8.

Clemente CD. Anatomy – a regional atlas of the human body. 4th ed. Baltimore: Williams and Wilkins; 1997.

Cruz J, Sousa J, Oliveira AG, Silva-Carvalho L. Effects of endoscopic thoracic sympathectomy for primary hyperhidrosis on cardiac autonomic nervous activity. J Thorac Cardiovasc Surg. 2009;137(3):664–9.

Fiorelli A, Vicidomini G, Laperuta P, Busiello L, Perrone A, Napolitano F, Messina G, Santini M. Pre-emptive local analgesia in video-assisted thoracic surgery sympathectomy. Eur J Cardiothorac Surg. 2010;37(3):588–93.

Freeman RK, Van Woerkom JM, Vyverberg A, Ascioti AJ. Reoperative endoscopic sympathectomy for persistent or recurrent palmar hyperhidrosis. Ann Thorac Surg. 2009;88(2):412–6. discussion 416–7.

Gardner PA, Ochalski PG, Moossy JJ. Minimally invasive endoscopic-assisted posterior thoracic sympathectomy. Neurosurg Focus. 2008;25(2):E6.

Jamieson GG. The anatomy of general surgical operations. 2nd ed. Edinburgh: Churchill Livingston; 2006.

Kim YD, Lee SH, Lee SY, Seo JH, Kim JJ, Sa YJ, Park CB, Kim CK, Moon SW, Yim HW. The effect of thoracosopic thoracic sympathetomy on pulmonary function and bronchial hyperresponsiveness. J Asthma. 2009;46(3):276–9.

Marhold F, Izay B, Zacherl J, Tschabitscher M, Neumayer C. Thoracoscopic and anatomic landmarks of Kuntz's nerve: implications for sympathetic surgery. Ann Thorac Surg. 2008; 86(5):1653–8.

Miller DL, Bryant AS, Force SD, Miller Jr JI. Effect of sympathectomy level on the incidence of compensatory hyperhidrosis after sympathectomy for palmar hyperhidrosis. J Thorac Cardiovasc Surg. 2009;138(3):581–5.

Rodríguez PM, Freixinet JL, Hussein M, Valencia JM, Gil RM, Herrero J, Caballero-Hidalgo A. Side effects, complications and outcome of thoracoscopic sympathectomy for palmar and axillary hyperhidrosis in 406 patients. Eur J Cardiothorac Surg. 2008;34(3):514–9.

Sabiston DC, Spencer FC. Surgery of the chest. 5th ed. Philadelphia: WB Saunders; 1990.

Shields TW. General thoracic surgery. 4th ed. Baltimore: Williams & Wilkins; 1994.

Sugimura H, Spratt EH, Compeau CG, Kattail D, Shargall Y. Thoracoscopic sympathetic clipping for hyperhidrosis: long-term results and reversibility. J Thorac Cardiovasc Surg. 2009;137(6): 1370–6. discussion 1376–7.

Weksler B, Blaine G, Souza ZB, Gavina R. Transection of more than one sympathetic chain ganglion for hyperhidrosis increases the severity of compensatory hyperhidrosis and decreases patient satisfaction. J Surg Res. 2009;156(1):110–5.

Westphal FL, de Campos JR, Ribas J, de Lima LC, Lima Netto JC, da Silva MS, Westphal DC. Skin depigmentation: could it be a complication caused by thoracic sympathectomy? Ann Thorac Surg. 2009;88(4):e42–3.

Yazbek G, Wolosker N, Kauffman P, de Campos JR, Puech-Leão P, Jatene FB. Twenty months of evolution following sympathectomy on patients with palmar hyperhidrosis: sympathectomy at the T3 level is better than at the T2 level. Clinics (Sao Paulo). 2009;64(8):743–9.

Chapter 4
Venous Surgery

David King, Robert Fitridge, John Walsh, and Brendon J. Coventry

Vascular Surgical Procedures General Perspective and Overview

The relative risks and complications increase proportionately according to the site of venous disease, within the vascular system. This is principally related to the surgical accessibility, ability to correct the problem, blood supply, risk of tissue injury, hematoma formation, and technical ease of surgery, including achieving an anastomosis when desired.

The main serious complications are **bleeding and infection,** which can be minimized by the adequate exposure, mobilization, reduction of tension, and ensuring satisfactory blood supply to the distal tissues. Infection is the main sequel of poor tissue perfusion or hematoma formation and may lead to **abscess formation** and **systemic sepsis**. **Multisystem failure** and **death** remain serious potential complications from vascular surgery and systemic infection.

D. King, BmedSc, MBBS, FRACS(GenSrg/Vasc) (✉)
Department of Vascular Surgery, Royal Adelaide Hospital,
Adelaide, Australia
e-mail: davidking@internode.on.net

R. Fitridge, MBBS, MS, FRACS
Discipline of Surgery, The Queen Elizabeth Hospital,
Woodville, Australia

J. Walsh, MD, FRACS
Discipline of Surgery, The Flinders University of South Australia,
Adelaide, Australia

B.J. Coventry, BMBS, PhD, FRACS, FACS, FRSM
Discipline of Surgery, Royal Adelaide Hospital, University of Adelaide,
L5 Eleanor Harrald Building, North Terrace,
5000 Adelaide, SA, Australia
e-mail: brendon.coventry@adelaide.edu.au

B.J. Coventry (ed.), *Cardio-Thoracic, Vascular, Renal and Transplant Surgery*,
Surgery: Complications, Risks and Consequences,
DOI 10.1007/978-1-4471-5418-1_4, © Springer-Verlag London 2014

Neural injuries are not infrequent potential problems associated with vascular surgery, because nerves commonly travel with vessels and are at risk of injury during dissection.

The risk of **bowel, bladder,** and **sexual dysfunction** increases with proximity to the pelvis and is almost exclusively associated with caval and iliac surgery.

Positioning on the operating table has been associated with increased risk of **deep venous thrombosis** and **nerve palsies,** especially in prolonged procedures. **Limb ischemia, compartment syndrome, and ulnar** and **common peroneal nerve palsy** are recognized potential complications, which should be checked for, as the patient's position may change during surgery.

Mortality associated with most venous vascular procedures is usually low and principally associated with pulmonary thromboembolism. Procedures involving the iliac veins or vena cava carry higher risks associated with possible serious bleeding and infection, including increased risk of mortality.

This chapter therefore attempts to draw together in one place the estimated overall frequencies of the complications associated with venous disease, based on information obtained from the literature and experience. Not all patients are at risk of the full range of listed complications. It must be individualized for each patient and their disease process, but represents a guide and summary of the attendant risks, complications, and consequences.

With these factors and facts in mind, the information given in this chapter must be appropriately and discernibly interpreted and used.

Important Note
It should be emphasized that the risks and frequencies that are given here *represent derived figures*. These *figures are best estimates of relative frequencies across most institutions*, not merely the highest-performing ones, and as such are often representative of a number of studies, which include different patients with differing comorbidities and different surgeons. In addition, the risks of complications in lower or higher risk patients may lie outside these estimated ranges, and individual clinical judgement is required as to the expected risks communicated to the patient or staff or for other purposes. The range of risks is also derived from experience and the literature; while risks outside this range may exist, certain risks may be reduced or absent due to variations of procedures or surgical approaches. It is recognized that different patients, practitioners, institutions, regions, and countries may vary in their requirements and recommendations.

For complications related to other associated/additional surgery that may arise during venous surgery, see the relevant volume and chapter.

Varicose Vein Surgery (High Saphenous Ligation + Stripping to Knee + Multiple Stab Avulsions of Varicosities): Primary or Secondary

Description

General or spinal anesthesia is usually used. Some pulling and movement of the patient can occur with the stripping of the long saphenous vein(s) (LSV). The aim is to remove the LSV if it is incompetent, using a vein stripping device, interrupt and ligate or strip any incompetent perforating veins between the deep and superficial venous systems, and interrupt superficial varicosities. This promotes flow through the deep system rather than reflux of blood into the incompetent superficial system, thus reducing the superficial varicosities and distension. Sometimes LSV high ligation at the saphenofemoral junction alone is performed, without stripping.

Anatomical Points

The saphenofemoral junction region is highly variable in the number and size of tributaries, but the location of the junction with the deep femoral vein is relatively constant being about 2–3 cm below and lateral to the pubic tubercle, well below the groin crease. A small arterial branch from the femoral artery typically travels medially between the long saphenous and femoral veins (across, anterior to, the femoral vein and posterior to the saphenous vein, just below the saphenofemoral junction) and is at risk of injury during dissection. Apart from the relatively constant long and short saphenous veins, the other superficial veins of the entire leg are highly variable. A communicating vein often exists between the long and short saphenous veins (Giacomini continuation). The saphenous nerve travels with the long saphenous vein below the knee and is at risk of injury from stripping the long saphenous vein below the knee.

Perspective

See Table 4.1. Varicose vein disease progression over time is usual, and therefore it is unclear whether development of some "complications or consequences" of varicose vein surgery is true "direct" results of the surgery or actually represents the "natural progression" of the underlying venous disease. Such complications or consequences as new varicose veins/spider veins/pain and discomfort/swelling/skin discoloration/ulceration and even DVT should be considered in this indeterminate

Table 4.1 Primary or secondary varicose vein surgery (HSL+stripping to knee) estimated frequency of complications, risks, and consequences

Complications, risks, and consequences	Estimated frequency
Most significant/serious complications	
Bleeding/bruising	>80 %
Hematoma formation	20–50 %
Infection	1–5 %
Nerve injury (overall)	1–5 %
Saphenous nerve (stripping to knee)	1–5 %
Sural nerve (short saphenous vein stripping)	1–5 %
Geniculate branches	0.1–1 %
Common peroneal	<0.1 %
Reformation of (significant) varicose veins	5–20 %
Rare significant/serious problems	
Swelling (major; leg/foot significant)	0.1–1 %
DVT (deep venous thrombosis)	0.1–1 %
PE (pulmonary embolus)	0.1–1 %
Stenosis of femoral vein (+/− thrombosis)	<0.1 %
Stripping superficial femoral artery/deep femoral vein[a]	<0.1 %
Less serious complications	
Swelling (minor; leg/foot significant)	1–5 %
Seroma/lymphocele formation	0.1–1 %
Residual pain/discomfort	1–5 %
Spider veins (development of)	5–20 %
Skin discoloration (long term)	1–5 %
Wound scarring (cosmetic)	1–5 %
Delayed wound healing (including ulceration)	1–5 %
Blood transfusion	<0.1 %

[a]Dependent on underlying pathology, anatomy, surgical technique, and preferences

category, which may potentially result from surgery. The other listed complications and risks are more clearly associated with surgery. Errors of femoral artery or deep femoral vein stripping, or stenosis of the femoral vein, are very rare and typically result from failure to adequately identify anatomic structures and represent extreme misadventure, perhaps related to inexperience. The incidence of saphenous nerve injury is directly related to stripping of the long saphenous vein below the knee where the nerve is closely applied to the vein. The risk of injury to the saphenous nerve can be effectively reduced, by only stripping of the long saphenous vein above the knee, where the nerve is separated from the vein. Saphenous nerve injury may occur during stab avulsions. Injury to any subcutaneous nerve or neural branch of the lower limb can result from incision and stab avulsion or injection sclerotherapy of varicosities or from ligation of perforators between the superficial and deep venous systems. Infection in the groin wounds is not uncommon and is usually associated with poor wound apposition, devitalization of the wound edges, hematoma formation, lymphocele, or wound separation. The infecting organisms are usually patient-derived endogenous cutaneous organisms such as staphylococci (*Staphylococcus aureus*) or gram-negative fecally derived organisms, e.g., *E. coli*, or a mixture of both. Preoperative prophylactic antibiotics should be given to cover both. The decision to prescribe prophylactic antibiotics remains an individual one. Seroma formation is not uncommon and leakage may occur. The relative patient satisfaction and acceptability of the risks can depend on the reason for surgery, whether for cosmetic improvement or for alleviation of venous congestion.

Major Complications

Severe bleeding intraoperatively or postoperatively is very rare, as is the resultant need for **blood transfusion**. Head-down (Trendelenburg) positioning usually reduces bleeding. **Severe bruising** may occur in some individuals, especially with impaired coagulation (iatrogenic or otherwise). **Injury to the femoral vein** (or artery) is rare and should be avoided with careful dissection, identification, and ligation of the saphenous vein at the saphenofemoral junction. **Infection** usually is avoided by using prophylactic antibiotics, but established infection can typically be treated with antibiotics and wound care. Major infections are rare except in immunocompromised individuals where special care and timing of surgery must be considered. Varicose vein surgery must be a balanced consideration and may need to be averted in these situations. **Severe damage to the femoral vein or artery** from stripping or direct ligation resulting from mistaken identity for the saphenous vein should be completely avoidable and not occur. **Deep venous thrombosis** and resultant pulmonary embolism are generally avoidable if adequate prophylaxis is used. Adequate ligation of blood vessels and lymphatics and judicious use of hemostatic diathermy are able to reduce risk of **large lymphocele, seroma, and hematoma**. **Major limb swelling** is unusual and avoidable by careful dissection and selective appropriate ligation of correct structures. Very rare severe swelling can result from atypical lymphatic interruption or obstruction from scarring. The use of bandages and graduated stockings often reduces the risk of swelling. Preexisting lymphatic drainage problems should be evaluated prior to varicose vein surgery and the patient adequately informed of the risk of potential worsening of limb swelling and possible permanency of this.

Consent and Risk Reduction

Main Points to Explain

- Discomfort
- Bleeding
- Recurrent varicosities
- DVT
- Infection
- Numbness
- Skin discoloration
- Scarring
- Further surgery
- Risks without surgery

Vena Cava Filter Surgery

Description

Local or general anesthesia can be used. Indications for IVC filters insertion are principally states of increased risk of PE, including DVT, recurrent PE, pelvic surgery, malignancy, major trauma, inability to anticoagulate effectively, and multiple fractures. Placement may be for prophylaxis in a high-risk situation or prevention of further embolic problems. Many caval filters are inserted currently by the percutaneous method by either radiologists or surgeons, which has largely replaced the traditional surgical insertions, but these are still sometimes performed. The aim is to place the caval filter, which is of several types, at the level of the inferior vena cava to prevent emboli, usually thrombotic, from further passage to the heart and pulmonary arterial circulation. The common type is the "umbrella type" filter that is inserted percutaneously collapsed within a sheath and is then expanded in the desired location in the IVC. The usual approach for insertion is via the femoral vein at the groin. Some designs can be removed after the danger period of pulmonary embolism has passed, and others are for permanent insertion.

Anatomical Points

The femoral vessels are relatively constant in their anatomy, as are the iliac vessels and IVC; however, venous duplication or differences in orientation with respect to the artery can occur at any level in the venous system. The superficial femoral vein is located medial to the femoral artery at the level of the groin, just medial to the midpoint of the inguinal ligament. Thrombosis of the femoral vein may render direct puncture difficult. Alternatively, filters can be inserted via the jugular and subclavian venous routes.

Perspective

See Table 4.2. Complications are relatively few in most cases; however, cases of serious complications including vena caval perforation, device malfunction, pulmonary embolism despite filter insertion, and migration, even intracardiac, are well reported, although fortunately relatively uncommon. Injury to any subcutaneous nerve can result from the groin, neck, or subclavicular insertion incision. Infection in the groin wounds can occur and is usually associated with poor wound apposition, devitalization of the wound edges, hematoma formation, lymphocele, seroma formation, or wound separation. Failure to place the IVC filter accurately can occur, as can thrombosis of the IVC. Preoperative prophylactic antibiotics are usually

Table 4.2 Vena cava filter surgery estimated frequency of complications, risks, and consequences

Complications, risks, and consequences	Estimated frequency
Most significant/serious complications	
Filter migration (late)[a]	5–20 %
Hematoma formation (groin or retroperitoneal)	1–5 %
Infection	1–5 %
Late device failure[a]	1–5 %
Vena caval obstruction	1–5 %
Rare significant/serious problems	
Early device malfunction/ineffective device deployment[a]	0.1–1 %
Vascular perforation	0.1–1 %
Pulmonary embolism	0.1–1 %
Femoral nerve injury	0.1–1 %
Seroma/lymphocele formation	0.1–1 %
Swelling (major; leg/foot significant)	0.1–1 %
DVT (deep venous thrombosis)	0.1–1 %
PE (pulmonary embolus)	0.1–1 %
Femoral arterial injury	0.1–1 %
Intracardiac filter migration[a]	<0.1 %
Open surgical filter extraction[a]	<0.1 %
Less serious complications	
Bleeding/bruising	20–50 %
Swelling (minor; leg/foot significant)	1–5 %
Delayed wound healing (including ulceration)	1–5 %
Blood transfusion	<0.1 %

[a]Dependent on underlying pathology, anatomy, surgical technique, and preferences

given. For removable devices, these are often inserted percutaneously via the femoral route and removed via the brachial or subclavian route.

Major Complications

Severe bleeding intraoperatively or postoperatively is very rare, as is the resultant need for **blood transfusion**. **Vena caval perforation** is very rare. **Severe bruising** may occur in some individuals, especially with impaired coagulation (iatrogenic or otherwise). **Injury to the femoral vein** (or artery) is rare and should be avoided with careful insertion/dissection. **Infection** usually is avoided by using prophylactic antibiotics and can typically be treated with antibiotics and wound care. Major infections are rare except in immunocompromised individuals where special care and timing of surgery must be considered. **Deep venous thrombosis** and resultant **pulmonary embolism** despite filter insertion is reported, either during device insertion, from clot forming above the in situ filter, or after device dislodgement. Risk of **large lymphocele, seroma, and hematoma** is relatively small. **Major limb swelling** is unusual, but severe phlegmasia cerulea dolens can occur. **Late device**

migration can occur in up to 10 % of cases. **Intracardiac filter migration** is very rare, but may require surgical extraction.

Consent and Risk Reduction

Main Points to Explain

- Discomfort
- Bleeding
- Recurrent embolism
- DVT
- Infection
- Filter migration
- Filter failure
- IVC perforation
- Further surgery
- Risks without surgery

Venous Injection Sclerotherapy Surgery

Description

Local or no anesthesia is often used. The aim is to induce local intravascular sclerosis with adhesion formation between the internal walls of the varicosities by injecting a sclerosing agents directly into the vessel, while limiting the washout of the injected agent, thereby concentrating the agent within the vessel for maximum fibrosis to occur. The fibrotic intravascular reaction aims to collapse and ablate the varicose segment of the superficial varicose vein(s). Several types of agents and several methods are used. Sodium tetradecyl sulfate and almond oil are commonly used sclerosing agents. The technique is principally for small- and medium sized varicosities. The washout effect of larger vessels and the relatively thicker wall make these less suitable and increase the risk of systemic reactions. Sclerotherapy can be used alone, after or combined simultaneously with venous stripping and avulsion.

Anatomical Points

The smaller tributaries of the saphenous vein and short saphenous vein are common sites for varicose veins. Communications between these and the deep venous

Table 4.3 Venous injection sclerotherapy estimated frequency of complications, risks, and consequences

Complications, risks, and consequences	Estimated frequency
Most significant/serious complications	
Bleeding/bruising	>80 %
Hematoma formation	20–50 %
Reformation of (significant) varicose veins	5–20 %
Infection	1–5 %
Nerve injury (overall)	1–5 %
Saphenous nerve (stripping to knee)	1–5 %
Sural nerve (short saphenous vein stripping)	1–5 %
Geniculate branches	0.1–1 %
Common peroneal	<0.1 %
Rare significant/serious problems	
Swelling (major; leg/foot significant)	0.1–1 %
DVT (deep venous thrombosis)	0.1–1 %
PE (pulmonary embolus)	0.1–1 %
Stenosis of femoral vein (+/− thrombosis)	<0.1 %
Stripping superficial femoral artery[a]	<0.1 %
Stripping deep femoral vein[a]	<0.1 %
Less serious complications	
Swelling (minor; leg/foot significant)	1–5 %
Seroma/lymphocele formation	0.1–1 %
Residual pain/discomfort	1–5 %
Spider veins (development of)	5–20 %
Skin discoloration (long term)	1–5 %
Wound scarring (cosmetic)	1–5 %
Delayed wound healing (including ulceration)	1–5 %
Blood transfusion	<0.1 %

[a]Dependent on underlying pathology, anatomy, surgical technique, and preferences

system, due to incompetent valves, cause superficial varicosities and "starburst" venous lesions, more common in the lower leg and foot. Reducing venous backflow may not always alleviate pressure and varicosities may persist or reform, at virtually any location in the lower limb. The saphenous nerve travels with the long saphenous vein below the knee and is at risk of injury from injection either directly or from the fibrotic reaction from the sclerosant.

Perspective

See Table 4.3. The procedure is largely performed for cosmetic reasons but may alleviate local pain from varicosities. Some local pain and discomfort may typically be experienced at the injection site(s) during injection of the sclerosant, local anesthetic, or both. Chronic pain is uncommon, but can occur. Varicose vein disease progression over time is usual, and therefore it is unclear whether development of some "complications or consequences" of varicose vein surgery is true direct results of any surgical procedure or actually represents the natural progression of the underlying venous disease. Such complications or consequences as new varicose veins/spider veins/pain and discomfort/swelling/skin discoloration/ulceration and even DVT should be considered in this indeterminate category, which may potentially result from surgery. The other listed complications and risks are more clearly associated with surgery. The incidence of saphenous nerve injury is directly related to injection close to of the long saphenous vein below the knee where the nerve is closely applied to the vein. Infection at the injection site(s), skin necrosis and ulceration, hematoma formation, or wound separation can occur. The infecting organisms are usually patient-derived endogenous cutaneous organisms such as staphylococci (*Staph. aureus*) or gram-negative fecally derived organisms, e.g., *E. coli*, or a mixture of both. Reformation of the varicosities, scarring, tenderness, bruising, skin discoloration, local swelling, and bleeding are common but typically settle within a month or so. DVT from the sclerosant entering the larger veins is rare.

Major Complications

Severe bleeding is very rare, but varicose veins that are subjected to high venous back pressure can bleed torrentially, if lacerated. **Severe bruising** may occur in some individuals, especially with impaired coagulation (iatrogenic or otherwise). **Injury to the femoral vein** (or artery) from the sclerosant is very rare but may induce **intravascular thrombosis** causing vessel occlusion. **Deep venous thrombosis**, although rare, is reported. **Infection** is unusual, but can occur, and may lead to **skin necrosis** and **ulceration**. Major infections are rare except in immunocompromised individuals where special care, timing, and the indications/wisdom of performing the procedure must be considered. Varicose vein injection sclerotherapy must be a balanced consideration and may need to be averted in these situations. **Major limb swelling** is very unusual, except when the underlying venous congestion worsens or DVT occurs. The use of bandages and graduated stockings often improves sclerosis and the results and reduces the risk of swelling. Preexisting lymphatic, venous, or arterial problems should be evaluated prior to varicose vein surgery of any type and requires the patient to be adequately informed of the risk of potential worsening of limb swelling and possible permanency of this. **Skin discoloration and scarring** may be considered a major complication by the patient, if cosmesis was the initial aim of the procedure.

Consent and Risk Reduction

Main Points to Explain

- Discomfort
- Bleeding
- Recurrent varicosities
- DVT
- Infection
- Skin discoloration
- Scarring
- Further surgery
- Risks without surgery

Further Reading, References, and Resources

Varicose Vein Surgery: Primary or Secondary

Bream E, Black N. What is the relationship between patients' and clinicians' reports of the outcomes of elective surgery? J Health Serv Res Policy. 2009;14(3):174–82. Review.

Clemente, CD. Anatomy – a regional atlas of the human body. 4th ed. Baltimore: Williams and Wilkins; 1997.

Darmas B. Should incompetent perforating veins surgery be a part of the surgical management of venous ulceration? Surgeon. 2009;7(4):238–42. Review.

Darwood RJ, Walker N, Bracey M, Cowan AR, Thompson JF, Campbell WB. Return to work, driving and other activities after varicose vein surgery is very variable and is influenced little by advice from specialists. Eur J Vasc Endovasc Surg. 2009;38(2):213–9.

Figueiredo M, Araújo S, Barros Jr N, Miranda Jr F. Results of surgical treatment compared with ultrasound-guided foam sclerotherapy in patients with Varicose Veins: a prospective randomised study. Eur J Vasc Endovasc Surg. 2009;38(6):758–63.

Jamieson GG. The anatomy of general surgical operations. 2nd ed. Edinburgh: Churchill Livingston; 2006.

Kouri B. Current evaluation and treatment of lower extremity varicose veins. Am J Med. 2009;122(6):513–5. Review.

Lewis DR. Who do you want to treat your varicose veins? N Z Med J. 2009;122(1295):61–4. Review.

Mouton WG, Keller S, Naef M, Wagner HE. Primary surgery for sapheno-femoral incompetence: a randomised controlled trial to compare two techniques to reduce lymphatic complications. Vasa. 2009;38(3):234–7.

Nishibe T, Kondo Y, Dardik A, Muto A, Nishibe M. Fate of varicose veins after great saphenous vein stripping alone. Int Angiol. 2009;28(4):311–4

O'Hare JL, Earnshaw JJ. Varicose veins today. Br J Surg. 2009;96(11):1229–30.

Parnaby CN, Welch GH, Stuart WP. An overview of the surgical aspects of lower limb venous disease. Scott Med J. 2009;54(3):30–5. Review.

Perkins JM. Standard varicose vein surgery. Phlebology. 2009;24 Suppl 1:34–41. Review.

Philipsen TE, De Maeseneer MG, Vandenbroeck CP, Van Schil PE. Anatomical patterns of the above knee great saphenous vein and its tributaries: implications for endovenous treatment strategy. Acta Chir Belg. 2009;109(2):176–9.

Pittaluga P, Chastanet S, Rea B, Barbe R. Midterm results of the surgical treatment of varices by phlebectomy with conservation of a refluxing saphenous vein. J Vasc Surg. 2009;50(1): 107–18.

Raju S, Neglén P. Clinical practice. Chronic venous insufficiency and varicose veins. N Engl J Med. 2009;360(22):2319–27. Review.

Theivacumar NS, Darwood R, Gough MJ. Neovascularisation and recurrence 2 years after varicose vein treatment for sapheno-femoral and great saphenous vein reflux: a comparison of surgery and endovenous laser ablation. Eur J Vasc Endovasc Surg. 2009;38(2):203.

van Neer P, Kessels FG, Estourgie RJ, de Haan EF, Neumann MA, Veraart JC. Persistent reflux below the knee after stripping of the great saphenous vein. J Vasc Surg. 2009;50(4):831–4.

Vena Cava Filter Surgery

Bogue CO, John PR, Connolly BL, Rea DJ, Amaral JG. Symptomatic caval penetration by a Celect inferior vena cava filter. Pediatr Radiol. 2009;39(10):1110–3.

Clemente CD. Anatomy – a regional atlas of the human body. 4th ed. Baltimore: Williams and Wilkins; 1997.

Corriere MA, Passman MA, Guzman RJ, Dattilo JB, Naslund TC. Retrieving "nonretrievable" inferior vena caval Greenfield filters: a therapeutic option for filter malpositioning. Ann Vasc Surg. 2004;18(6):629–34.

Corriere MA, Piercy KT, Edwards MS. Vena cava filters: an update. Future Cardiol. 2006;2(6): 695–707.

De Gregorio MA, Gamboa P, Bonilla DL, Sanchez M, Higuera MT, Medrano J, Mainar A, Lostalé F, Laborda A. Retrieval of Gunther Tulip optional vena cava filters 30 days after implantation: a prospective clinical study. J Vasc Interv Radiol. 2006;17(11 Pt 1):1781–9.

Gaspard SF, Gaspard DJ. Retrievable inferior vena cava filters are rarely removed. Am Surg. 2009;75(5):426–8.

Given MF, McDonald BC, Brookfield P, Niggemeyer L, Kossmann T, Varma DK, Thomson KR, Lyon SM. Retrievable Gunther Tulip inferior vena cava filter: experience in 317 patients. J Med Imaging Radiat Oncol. 2008;52(5):452–7.

Goldhaber SZ. Advanced treatment strategies for acute pulmonary embolism, including thrombolysis and embolectomy. J Thromb Haemost. 2009;7 Suppl 1:322–7.

Jamieson GG. The anatomy of general surgical operations. 2nd ed. Edinburgh: Churchill Livingston; 2006.

Joels CS, Sing RF, Heniford BT. Complications of inferior vena cava filters. Am Surg. 2003;69(8):654–9. Review.

Johnson 3rd ON, Gillespie DL, Aidinian G, White PW, Adams E, Fox CJ. The use of retrievable inferior vena cava filters in severely injured military trauma patients. J Vasc Surg. 2009;49(2):410–6. discussion 416.

Keeling WB, Haines K, Stone PA, Armstrong PA, Murr MM, Shames ML. Current indications for preoperative inferior vena cava filter insertion in patients undergoing surgery for morbid obesity. Obes Surg. 2005;15(7):1009–12.

Keeling AN, Kinney TB, Lee MJ. Optional inferior vena caval filters: where are we now? Eur Radiol. 2008;18(8):1556–68.

Lam RC, Bush RL, Lin PH, Lumsden AB. Early technical and clinical results with retrievable inferior vena caval filters. Vascular. 2004;12(4):233–7.

Nazzal M, Abbas J, Shattu J, Nazzal M. Complications secondary to the Bard retrievable filter: a case report. Ann Vasc Surg. 2008;22(5):684–7.

Parkin E, Serracino-Inglott F, Chalmers N, Smyth V. Symptomatic perforation of a retrievable inferior vena cava filter after a dwell time of 5 years. J Vasc Surg. 2009;50(2):417–9.

Saour J, Al Harthi A, El Sherif M, Bakhsh E, Mammo L. Inferior vena caval filters: 5 years of experience in a tertiary care center. Ann Saudi Med. 2009;29(6): 446–9.

Uppal B, Flinn WR, Benjamin ME. The bedside insertion of inferior vena cava filters using ultrasound guidance. Perspect Vasc Surg Endovasc Ther. 2007;19(1):78–84.

Usoh F, Hingorani A, Ascher E, Shiferson A, Tran V, Marks N, Jacob T. Long-term follow-up for superior vena cava filter placement. Ann Vasc Surg. 2009;23(3):350–4.

Venous Injection Sclerotherapy

Al Samaraee A, McCallum IJ, Mudawi A. Endovenous therapy of varicose veins: a better outcome than standard surgery? Surgeon. 2009;7(3):181–6. Review.

Bachoo P. Interventions for uncomplicated varicose veins. Phlebology. 2009;24 Suppl 1:3–12. Review.

Chapman-Smith P, Browne A. Prospective five-year study of ultrasound-guided foam sclerotherapy in the treatment of great saphenous vein reflux. Phlebology. 2009;24(4):183–8.

Clemente CD. Anatomy – a regional atlas of the human body. 4th ed. Baltimore: Williams and Wilkins; 1997.

Darvall KA, Bate GR, Silverman SH, Adam DJ, Bradbury AW. Medium-term results of ultrasound-guided foam sclerotherapy for small saphenous varicose veins. Br J Surg. 2009;96(11): 1268–73.

Goode SD, Kuhan G, Altaf N, Simpson R, Beech A, Richards T, MacSweeney ST, Braithwaite BD. Suitability of varicose veins for endovenous treatments. Cardiovasc Intervent Radiol. 2009;32(5):988–91.

Hamel-Desnos CM, Gillet JL, Desnos PR, Allaert FA. Sclerotherapy of varicose veins in patients with documented thrombophilia: a prospective controlled randomized study of 105 cases. Phlebology. 2009;24(4):176–82.

Jamieson GG. The anatomy of general surgical operations. 2nd ed. Edinburgh: Churchill Livingston; 2006.

Lewis DR. Who do you want to treat your varicose veins? N Z Med J. 2009;122(1295):61–4. Review.

Nael R, Rathbun S. Effectiveness of foam sclerotherapy for the treatment of varicose veins. Vasc Med. 2010;15(1):27–32.

Nishibe T, Kondo Y, Dardik A, Muto A, Nishibe M. Fate of varicose veins after great saphenous vein stripping alone. Int Angiol. 2009;28(4):311–4.

Wright DD, Gibson KD, Barclay J, Razumovsky A, Rush J, McCollum CN. High prevalence of right-to-left shunt in patients with symptomatic great saphenous incompetence and varicose veins. J Vasc Surg. 2010;51(1):104–7.

Chapter 5
Amputation Surgery

Brendon J. Coventry and John Walsh

General Perspective and Overview

The relative risks and complications increase proportionately according to the site and nature of vascular disease, trauma, or amputation. This is principally related to the vascular supply, surgical accessibility, ability to correct the problem, risk of tissue/organ injury, hematoma formation, and technical ease of surgery, including achieving adequate cover of bone and nerve tissue.

The main serious complications are **bleeding, infection, and wound breakdown,** which can be minimized by the adequate planning, exposure, mobilization, reduction of tension, and ensuring satisfactory blood supply to the tissues. Infection is the main sequel of poor tissue perfusion or hematoma formation and may lead to **abscess formation** and **systemic sepsis. Multisystem failure** and **death** remain serious potential complications from amputation surgery and systemic infection, especially in elderly individuals with ischemic preexisting tissues.

Neural injuries are not infrequent potential problems associated with amputation surgery, because nerves commonly travel with vessels and are at risk of injury during dissection. **Neuroma formation**, especially at the limb stump, can be problematic.

Positioning on the operating table has been associated with increased risk of **deep venous thrombosis** and **nerve palsies**, especially in prolonged procedures. **Limb ischemia, compartment syndrome, and ulnar** and **common peroneal**

B.J. Coventry, BMBS, PhD, FRACS, FACS, FRSM (✉)
Discipline of Surgery, Royal Adelaide Hospital, University of Adelaide,
L5 Eleanor Harrald Building, North Terrace, 5000 Adelaide, SA, Australia
e-mail: brendon.coventry@adelaide.edu.au

J. Walsh, MD, FRACS
Discipline of Surgery, The Flinders University of South Australia, Adelaide, Australia

B.J. Coventry (ed.), *Cardio-Thoracic, Vascular, Renal and Transplant Surgery*,
Surgery: Complications, Risks and Consequences,
DOI 10.1007/978-1-4471-5418-1_5, © Springer-Verlag London 2014

nerve palsy are recognized potential complications, which should be checked for, as the patient's position may change during surgery.

Mortality associated with amputation procedures ranges from <0.1 % for simple procedures up to >80 % overall (30-day perioperative mortality) for individual urgent complex high-risk amputations. Variation of this type is well recognized and relatively common, depending on the underlying disease, type of procedure, and the extent of comorbidities, which needs to be taken into account when assessing risk or interpreting data.

This chapter therefore attempts to draw together in one place the estimated overall frequencies of the complications associated with amputation, based on information obtained from the literature and experience. Not all patients are at risk of the full range of listed complications. It must be individualized for each patient and their disease process but represents a guide and summary of the attendant risks, complications, and consequences.

With these factors and facts in mind, the information given in this chapter must be appropriately and discernibly interpreted and used.

The **use of specialized units with standardized preoperative assessment, multidisciplinary input, and high-quality postoperative care, especially rehabilitation care,** is essential to the success of amputation surgery overall and significantly reduces risk of complications, recovery, and cost. **Mobilization postamputation** may be limited by the exercise capacity from comorbidities, such as cardiovascular or lung disease, where using crutches demands up to 300 % more energy than usual walking.

Important Note

It should be emphasized that the risks and frequencies that are given here *represent derived figures. These figures are best estimates of relative frequencies across most institutions*, not merely the highest-performing ones, and as such are often representative of a number of studies, which include different patients with differing comorbidities and different surgeons. In addition, the risks of complications in lower- or higher-risk patients may lie outside these estimated ranges, and individual clinical judgement is required as to the expected risks communicated to the patient, staff, or for other purposes. The range of risks is also derived from experience and the literature; while risks outside this range may exist, certain risks may be reduced or absent due to variations of procedures or surgical approaches. It is recognized that different patients, practitioners, institutions, regions, and countries may vary in their requirements and recommendations.

For complications related to other associated/additional surgery that may arise during amputation surgery, see the relevant chapter, for example, Arterial Surgery (Chap. 3).

Above-Knee Amputation

Description

General anesthesia is usually preferable; however, spinal, regional, or local anesthesia can be used. The aim is to remove the lower limb above the knee joint, usually through the lower 1/3 of the femur, although this is dependent on the pathology. The usual indications are necrosis, irreversible ischemia, trauma, tumor, or lack of function of the distal lower limb, not amenable to below-knee amputation. Preservation of the knee is preferable, using below-knee amputation, if feasible. Skin and muscle flaps are fashioned anteriorly and posteriorly, retaining as much usable tissue as practicable. The femur is cut, trimmed, and shaped to reduce tissue trauma from the bone end, and the vessels and nerves are ligated as high as possible above the end of the femur to prevent injury to these during postoperative mobilization. Typically, relatively equal skin flaps are sutured together loosely over the femoral bone end.

Anatomical Points

The anatomy of the lower limb is relatively constant; however, the underlying disease process and the surrounding tissue viability may dictate the type and precise level of amputation. The integrity of the other limb is very important in determining mobility.

Perspective

See Table 5.1. Minor complications are relatively common; however, most of these will usually settle with dressings and antibiotics. These include minor bleeding, oozing, superficial infection, swelling, numbness, minor ulceration, minor dehiscence, and discomfort. Major complications can occur and include osteomyelitis, severe hemorrhage from a slipped femoral arterial ligature, complete wound dehiscence, keloid scarring, and muscle necrosis, all of which may require further

Table 5.1 Above-knee amputation estimated frequency of complications, risks, and consequences

Complications, risks, and consequences	Estimated frequency
Most significant/serious complications	
Infection (overall)	1–5 %
Wound	1–5 %
Bone associated (osteomyelitis)	0.1–1 %
Systemic sepsis	0.1–1 %

(continued)

Table 5.1 (continued)

Complications, risks, and consequences	Estimated frequency
Bleeding or hematoma formation	
Wound	1–5 %
False aneurysm	0.1–1 %
Arteriovenous fistula	0.1–1 %
Muscle necrosis	1–5 %
Flap necrosis	5–20 %
Rare significant/serious problems	
Bone protuberance	0.1–1 %
Deep venous thrombosis/pulmonary embolus	0.1–1 %
Verrucous change chronic edema	0.1–1 %
Chronic wound dressings	0.1–1 %
Gas gangrene/necrotizing fasciitis	<0.1 %
Mortality[a]	<0.1 %
Less serious complications	
Residual pain/discomfort/tenderness	
Short term (<4 weeks)	50–80 %
Longer term (>12 weeks)	0.1–1 %
Fat necrosis	1–5 %
Pressure necrosis	5–20 %
Pressure ulcers	1–5 %
Stump neuroma	1–5 %
Pressure hypertrophy	1–5 %
Wound dehiscence	1–5 %
Seroma/lymphatic fluid leak/lymphocele formation	1–5 %
Mobilization balance problems	50–80 %
Forgetting amputation during mobilization	50–80 %
Phantom pain	50–80 %
Phantom limb	50–80 %
Delayed wound healing (including ulceration)	5–20 %
Wound scarring (poor cosmesis)	5–20 %

[a]Dependent on underlying pathology, anatomy, surgical technique, and preferences

surgery or other treatment, including antibiotics. Mobility typically becomes more problematic the higher the amputation is on the limb.

Major Complications

Perhaps the most serious complications after amputation are **severe bleeding**, **complete wound dehiscence**, and **serious infections**, including **osteomyelitis**. **Mobility problems** can also cause serious chronic disability. **Flap necrosis** and **infection** can also cause considerable problems and rarely result in **systemic infection, necrotizing infections,** and even **multisystem organ failure**, especially in elderly patients, diabetics, and with other comorbidities. **Chronic pain** can also be a major problem and reduce mobility.

Consent and Risk Reduction

Main Points to Explain

- Discomfort/pain
- Bleeding
- Poor function
- Infection
- Stiffness
- Poor mobilization

Below-Knee Amputation

Description

General anesthesia is usually preferable; however, spinal, regional, or local anesthesia can be used. The aim is to remove the lower limb below the knee joint, usually through the upper 1/3 of the lower limb, although this is dependent on the pathology. The usual indications are necrosis, irreversible ischemia, trauma, tumor, or loss of function of the distal lower limb, not amenable to lower amputation. Preservation of the knee aids locomotion greatly. Skin and muscle flaps are fashioned anteriorly and posteriorly, retaining as much usable tissue as practicable. The tibia and fibula are cut, trimmed, and shaped to reduce tissue trauma from the bone ends, and the vessels and nerves are ligated as high as possible above the bone ends to prevent injury to these during post-operative mobilization. The fibula is cut shorter than the tibia. Typically, the posterior skin flap with the calf muscles is retained longer than the anterior flap, to enable the posterior flap to be brought over the bone ends and sutured more anteriorly.

Anatomical Points

The anatomy of the lower limb is relatively constant; however, the underlying disease process may dictate the type and precise level of amputation. The integrity of the other limb is very important in determining mobility.

Perspective

See Table 5.2. Minor complications are relatively common; however, most of these will usually settle with dressings and antibiotics. These include minor bleeding, oozing, superficial infection, swelling, numbness, minor ulceration, minor dehiscence, and discomfort. Major complications can occur and include osteomyelitis,

Table 5.2 Below-knee amputation estimated frequency of complications, risks, and consequences

Complications, risks, and consequences	Estimated frequency
Most significant/serious complications	
Infection (overall)	5–20 %
Wound	5–20 %
Bone associated (osteomyelitis)	0.1–1 %
Systemic sepsis	0.1–1 %
Bleeding or hematoma formation	
Wound	1–5 %
False aneurysm	0.1–1 %
Arteriovenous fistula	0.1–1 %
Muscle necrosis	1–5 %
Flap necrosis	5–20 %
Pressure ulcers	1–5 %
Rare significant/serious problems	
Bone protuberance	0.1–1 %
Deep venous thrombosis/pulmonary embolus	0.1–1 %
Gas gangrene/necrotizing fasciitis	<0.1 %
Mortality[a]	<0.1 %
Less serious complications	
Fat necrosis	1–5 %
Wound dehiscence	1–5 %
Seroma/lymphocele formation	1–5 %
Stump neuroma	5–20 %
Pressure necrosis	5–20 %
Pressure hypertrophy	1–5 %
Residual pain/discomfort	1–5 %
Lymphatic fluid leak	1–5 %
Mobilization balance problems	>80 %
Forgetting amputation during mobilization	50–80 %
Phantom pain	50–80 %
Phantom limb	50–80 %
Verrucous change chronic edema	0.1–1 %
Delayed wound healing (including ulceration)	5–20 %
Wound scarring (poor cosmesis)	5–20 %

[a]Dependent on underlying pathology, anatomy, surgical technique, and preferences

septic arthritis of the knee, severe hemorrhage from a slipped arterial ligature, complete wound dehiscence, keloid scarring, and muscle necrosis, all of which may require further surgery or other treatment, including antibiotics. Mobility typically becomes more problematic the higher the amputation is on the limb.

Major Complications

Perhaps the most serious complications after amputation are **severe bleeding, complete wound dehiscence,** and **serious infections**, including **osteomyelitis** and

septic arthritis. Mobility problems can also cause serious disability. **Flap necrosis** and **infection** can also cause considerable problems and rarely result in **systemic infection, necrotizing infections,** and even **multisystem organ failure**, especially in elderly patients, diabetics, and with other comorbidities. **Chronic pain** can also be a major problem and reduce mobility.

Consent and Risk Reduction

Main Points to Explain

- Discomfort/pain
- Bleeding
- Poor function
- Infection
- Stiffness
- Poor mobilization

Digital Amputation Traumatic or Elective

Description

General anesthesia is usually preferable; however, spinal, regional, or local anesthesia can be used. The aim is to remove the digit through the bone or joint suitably above the site of the pathology, although this is dependent on the exact pathology. The usual indications are trauma, necrosis, irreversible ischemia, tumor, or loss of function of the digit, not amenable to other treatments. Preservation of a joint aids locomotion greatly. Skin and muscle flaps are fashioned anteriorly and posteriorly, retaining as much usable tissue as practicable. The bone shaft or joint is cut, trimmed, and shaped to reduce tissue trauma from the bone end, and the vessels and nerves are ligated as high as possible above the bone ends to prevent injury to these during postoperative mobilization and use. The skin flaps are sutured together over the bone end, often with one flap longer to wrap the skin over the bone, placing the suture line away from the bone end. It is often preferable to protect the volar surface of the finger/thumb or toe with a thicker flap to cushion the bone against pressure during use.

Anatomical Points

The anatomy of the digit is relatively constant; however, the underlying disease process may dictate the type and precise level of amputation. The integrity of the other digits and limb is very important in determining mobility.

Table 5.3 Digital amputation estimated frequency of complications, risks, and consequences

Complications, risks, and consequences	Estimated frequency
Most significant/serious complications	
Infection (overall)	1–5 %
Wound	1–5 %
Bone associated (osteomyelitis)[a]	0.1–1 %
Systemic sepsis	0.1–1 %
Bleeding or hematoma Formation	
Wound	1–5 %
Muscle necrosis[a]	1–5 %
Bone protuberance[a]	0.1–1 %
Flap necrosis	5–20 %
Rare significant/serious problems	
Pressure necrosis	0.1–1 %
Gas gangrene/necrotizing fasciitis	<0.1 %
Less serious complications	
Pressure ulcers	0.1–1 %
Fat necrosis	1–5 %
Wound dehiscence	1–5 %
Seroma/lymphocele formation	1–5 %
Residual pain/discomfort	1–5 %
Stump neuroma[a]	1–5 %
Phantom pain	50–80 %
Phantom digit	50–80 %
Delayed wound healing (including ulceration)[a]	1–5 %
Wound scarring (poor cosmesis)	5–20 %

[a]Dependent on underlying pathology, anatomy, surgical technique, and preferences

Perspective

See Table 5.3. Minor complications are relatively common; however, most of these will usually settle with dressings and antibiotics. These include minor bleeding, oozing, superficial infection, swelling, numbness, minor ulceration, minor dehiscence, and discomfort. Major complications can occur and include osteomyelitis, septic arthritis of an adjacent joint, hemorrhage from a slipped arterial ligature, complete wound dehiscence, keloid scarring, and muscle necrosis, all of which may require further surgery or other treatment, including antibiotics. Mobility and function typically become more problematic the higher the amputation is on the digit.

Major Complications

Perhaps the most serious complications after amputation are **severe bleeding, complete wound dehiscence,** and **serious infections,** including **osteomyelitis** and

septic arthritis. Mobility problems can also cause serious disability. **Flap necrosis** and **infection** can also cause considerable problems and rarely result in **systemic infection, necrotizing infections,** and even rarely **multisystem organ failure**, especially in elderly patients, diabetics, and with other comorbidities. **Chronic pain** can also be a major problem and reduce mobility.

Consent and Risk Reduction

Main Points to Explain

- Discomfort/pain
- Bleeding
- Poor function
- Infection
- Stiffness

Further Reading, References, and Resources

Above-Knee Amputation

Clemente CD. Anatomy – a regional atlas of the human body. 4th ed. Baltimore: Williams and Wilkins; 1997.

Jamieson GG. The anatomy of general surgical operations. 2nd ed. Edinburgh: Churchill Livingston; 2006.

Below-Knee Amputation

Clemente CD. Anatomy – a regional atlas of the human body. 4th ed. Baltimore: Williams and Wilkins; 1997.

Jamieson GG. The anatomy of general surgical operations. 2nd ed. Edinburgh: Churchill Livingston; 2006.

Digital Amputation

Clemente CD. Anatomy – a regional atlas of the human body. 4th ed. Baltimore: Williams and Wilkins; 1997.

Clebes F, Fuchs FD, Fagundes A, Poerschke RA, Vacaro MZ. Prognostic factors for amputation or death in patients submitted to vascular surgery for acute limb ischemia. Vasc Health Risk Manag. 2005;1(4):345–9.

Goodney PP, Travis LL, Nallamothu BK, Holman K, Suckow B, Henke PK, Lucas FL, Goodman DC, Birkmeyer JD, Fisher ES. Variation in the use of lower extremity vascular procedures for critical limb ischemia. Circ Cardiovasc Qual Outcomes. Author manuscript; available in PMC 2013 Jan 1. Published in final edited form as: Circ Cardiovasc Qual Outcomes. 2012;5(1): 94–102.

Jamieson GG. The anatomy of general surgical operations. 2nd ed. Edinburgh: Churchill Livingston; 2006.

Simons JP, Schanzer A, Nolan BW, Stone DH, Kalish JA, Cronenwett JL, Goodney PP. A Contemporary analysis of outcomes and practice patterns in patients undergoing lower extremity bypass in New England. J Vasc Surg. Author manuscript; available in PMC 2013 June 1. Published in final edited form as: J Vasc Surg. 2012;55(6):1629–36.

Suckow BD, Goodney PP, Cambria RA, Bertges DJ, Eldrup-Jorgensen J, Indes JE, Schanzer A, Stone DH, Kraiss LW, Cronenwett JL. Predicting functional status following amputation after lower extremity bypass Ann Vasc Surg. Author manuscript; available in PMC 2012 April 30. Published in final edited form as: Ann Vasc Surg. 2012;26(1):67–78.

Venermo M, Manderbacka K, Ikonen T, Keskimäki I, Winell K, Sund R. Amputations and socioeconomic position among persons with diabetes mellitus, a population-based register study. BMJ Open. 2013;3(4):e002395.

Ziegler KR, Muto A, Eghbalieh SDD, Dardik A. Basic data related to operative infrainguinal revascularization procedures: a twenty year update. Ann Vasc Surg. Author manuscript; available in PMC 2012 April 1. Published in final edited form as: Ann Vasc Surg. 2011;25(3): 413–22.

Chapter 6
Vascular Access Surgery

Christine Russell, David King, and Brendon J. Coventry

General Perspective and Overview

The relative risks and complications increase proportionately according to the site and size of the vessel being accessed within the vascular system. This is principally related to the surgical accessibility, ability to cannulate, risk of laceration or tissue injury, hematoma formation, and technical ease, including achieving patency and flow of the infusate.

The main serious complications are **bleeding and infection,** which can be minimized by the adequate exposure, mobilization, technical care, and ensuring direct entry of needles and catheters into the vessel lumen to avoid laceration and hematoma formation. Infection is the main sequel of tissue injury and hematoma formation and may arise from skin organisms especially with long-term indwelling percutaneous catheterization. This can lead to **abscess formation** and **systemic sepsis**. **Multisystem failure** and **death** remain serious potential complications from vascular access (device) surgery and systemic infection.

Neural injuries are not infrequent potential problems associated with vascular access surgery, because nerves commonly travel with or across vessels and are at risk of injury during percutaneous puncture or dissection.

C. Russell, BA, BM BCh FRACS (✉)
Central and Northern Adelaide Renal and Transplantation Service,
Royal Adelaide Hospital, Adelaide, Australia
e-mail: christine.russell3@health.sa.gov.au

D. King, BmedSc, MBBS, FRACS(GenSrg/Vasc)
Department of Vascular Surgery, Royal Adelaide Hospital, Adelaide, Australia

B.J. Coventry, BMBS, PhD, FRACS, FACS, FRSM
Discipline of Surgery, Royal Adelaide Hospital, University of Adelaide,
L5 Eleanor Harrald Building, North Terrace, 5000 Adelaide, SA, Australia
e-mail: brendon.coventry@adelaide.edu.au

B.J. Coventry (ed.), *Cardio-Thoracic, Vascular, Renal and Transplant Surgery*,
Surgery: Complications, Risks and Consequences,
DOI 10.1007/978-1-4471-5418-1_6, © Springer-Verlag London 2014

Positioning on the operating table has been associated with increased risk of **deep venous thrombosis** and **nerve palsies**, especially in prolonged procedures. **Limb ischemia, compartment syndrome, and ulnar** and **common peroneal nerve palsy** are recognized potential complications, which should be checked for, as the patient's position may change during surgery. Most vascular access surgery is brief, and risks of positioning injuries are therefore usually lessened.

Mortality associated with most venous vascular access procedures is usually low and principally associated with pulmonary thromboembolism or catheter or vessel thrombosis or occlusion. Procedures involving the iliac veins or vena cava or larger arteries carry higher risks associated with possible serious bleeding and infection, including increased risk of mortality.

This chapter therefore attempts to draw together in one place, the estimated overall frequencies of the complications associated with vascular access procedures, based on information obtained from the literature and experience. Not all patients are at risk of the full range of listed complications. It must be individualized for each patient and their disease process but represents a guide and summary of the attendant risks, complications, and consequences.

With these factors and facts in mind, the information given in this chapter must be appropriately and discernibly interpreted and used.

Important Note

It should be emphasized that the risks and frequencies that are given here *represent derived figures. These figures are best estimates of relative frequencies across most institutions*, not merely the highest-performing ones, and as such are often representative of a number of studies, which include different patients with differing comorbidities and different surgeons. In addition, the risks of complications in lower- or higher-risk patients may lie outside these estimated ranges, and individual clinical judgement is required as to the expected risks communicated to the patient, staff, or for other purposes. The range of risks is also derived from experience and the literature; while the risks outside this range may exist, certain risks may be reduced or absent due to variations of procedures or surgical approaches. It is recognized that different patients, practitioners, institutions, regions, and countries may vary in their requirements and recommendations.

For complications related to other associated/additional surgery that may arise during vascular access surgery, see Chap. 3 Arterial Surgery or Chap. 4 Venous Surgery or the relevant volume and chapter.

Central Venous Catheter Line Insertion

Description

Local anesthesia is usually well tolerated and preferable in adults; however, general anesthesia may be used on occasions. The aim is to gain access to the subclavian or internal jugular vein by direct puncture using a percutaneous Seldinger technique (guidewire, dilator, separable sheath, Silastic catheter). Once inserted into the vein, the sheath can be stripped away, leaving the venous catheter. The position of the catheter in the superior vena cava can then be checked using image intensification radiology. Alternatively, an open approach can be used, although this is more traumatic to the vein and is generally reserved for situations where percutaneous access is difficult or inadvisable. The skin puncture rarely requires closure, and usually a waterproof dressing is all that is needed. Occasionally, a more peripheral vein is used (e.g., cephalic) or a groin approach to the femoral/iliac vein and inferior vena cava for central vein access, but these are not considered further here, although many of the complications that can arise are similar.

Anatomical Points

The position of the subclavian and internal jugular veins is relatively constant; however, there is some relative minor variation due to differences in the surrounding bony anatomy between individuals and the hydration status of the patient. Dehydration decreases venous size and can make access more difficult. Placing the patient slightly "head-down" is also helpful in dilating the venous system of the head and neck facilitating easier entry of the initial needle and reduces risk of air embolism. The pleura lies behind the medial 1/3 of the clavicle on each side and is at risk of puncture and inducing a pneumothorax.

Perspective

See Table 6.1. The procedure is usually associated with a low complication rate and most are minor, such as bruising, difficulty gaining access to the vein, and minor superficial infection. Major complications are rare but can occur, such as pneumothorax, which may require further hospitalization or insertion of an underwater-seal chest drain tube. Cardiac arrhythmias and bleeding are risks during insertion. Immediate withdrawal of the catheter wire or tube several centimeters will usually

Table 6.1 Central venous line insertion estimated frequency of complications, risks, and consequences

Complications, risks, and consequences	Estimated frequency
Most significant/serious complications	
Infection (overall)[a]	5–20 %
Wound	5–20 %
Within the catheter	5–20 %
Systemic sepsis	1–5 %
Bleeding/hematoma formation[a] (wound)	1–5 %
Thrombosis – SVC thrombosis/internal jugular/cephalic vein	1–5 %
Migration/displacement of the catheter tube	1–5 %
Catheter failure (from whatever cause) [misdirection, occlusion, kinking, fracture/breakage, too long/short]	1–5 %
Rare significant/serious problems	
Nerve injury (depending on positioning) [cutaneous nerve, Vagus X nerve damage, etc.]	0.1–1 %
Pneumothorax	0.1–1 %
Failure to perform catheter insertion (technical problems)	0.1–1 %
Catheter tip embolus	0.1–1 %
Cardiac arrhythmias (catheter irritation of endocardium)	0.1–1 %
Catheter or guidewire vascular perforation[a]	<0.1 %
Cardiac perforation and tamponade[a]	<0.1 %
Subclavian vein fistula	<0.1 %
Hemothorax	<0.1 %
Air embolism	<0.1 %
Multisystem organ failure[a]	<0.1 %
Death[a]	<0.1 %
Less serious complications	
Bruising	20–50 %
Residual pain/discomfort/neuralgia	1–5 %
Radiation exposure (for the patient) (low level)	>80 %
Wound dehiscence	1–5 %
Skin/fat necrosis	0.1–1 %
Delayed wound healing (including ulceration)	1–5 %
Wound scarring (poor cosmesis)	1–5 %

[a]Dependent on underlying pathology, anatomy, surgical technique, preferences, and comorbidities

settle the arrhythmia. Catheter thrombosis, cardiac arrhythmias, and migration of the catheter are also potentially serious as the catheter may require removal and later reinsertion. Catheter or guidewire perforation of vessels or the heart is very rare, but both are well reported, but these have been almost "designed out" with soft-ended devices. Percutaneous CVC lines invariably fail over time due to infection, mechanical problems, or thrombosis, and regular replacement may avert these issues as clinical complications. Failure to complete the procedure by the percutaneous method will not usually disallow its insertion, since the open approach can usually then be used. Bilateral attempts at central line insertion via the subclavian approach are not advisable within 24 h of each other, as there is a risk of inducing bilateral pneumothoraces. Use of the internal jugular approach is preferable after a failed subclavian approach to reduce pneumothorax risk.

Major Complications

The main severe acute complications are **pneumothorax, cardiac arrhythmias, air embolism,** and **hemothorax.** Later, **infection** of the catheter line can lead to **systemic sepsis** and even **multisystem organ failure**, which is the major cause of **mortality**, especially in immunocompromised patients and severely ill patients. **Catheter tip bacterial colonization or thrombosis** with consequent **embolization** of material can occur and may be associated with bacterial endocarditis, metastatic infection, or pulmonary embolism. **Removal of the central line** invariably follows infection. Air embolism and hemothorax are very rare but can be life-threatening. **Catheter blockage or leakage** due to a variety of problems may require removal and reinsertion or adjustment. **Catheter thrombosis** and **pulmonary embolism** can occur and may be serious. **Axillary, subclavian, internal jugular, or superior vena cava venous** thrombosis can cause severe swelling of the arm, neck, head, and chest. **Carotid artery puncture** is minimized by the use of ultrasound guidance. **Cardiac arrhythmias** are usually terminated by withdrawal of the guidewire from the heart chamber, usually the atrium affecting the sinoatrial node. **Catheter tip migration** can occur into the jugular vein, opposite subclavian vein, right heart, IVC, or even pulmonary artery. **Catheter or guidewire vascular perforation** is very rare, especially with J-hooked, soft-tipped guidewires or soft catheters, but both are well reported. **Cardiac perforation and tamponade** is exceedingly rare. **Catheter fracture and embolism** is reported and may require radiological or rarely open surgical removal.

Consent and Risk Reduction

Main Points to Explain

- Discomfort
- Bruising and bleeding
- Infection
- Pneumothorax (rare)
- Cardiac arrhythmias (usually minor)
- Failure of insertion
- Catheter displacement/later failure
- Further surgery

Tunneled Internal Jugular Central Venous Catheter Line Insertion

Description

Local anesthesia or general anesthesia may be used. The line can be inserted percutaneously or via an open approach. The aim is to insert the catheter into the subclavian or internal jugular vein percutaneously (or open) and to tunnel this subcutaneously to a convenient site in the anterior axilla, upper chest, or abdomen for exit and access. The line can be inserted percutaneously or via an open approach. If using the percutaneous route, the use of ultrasound guidance may lower the complication rate. It is important to measure the catheter so that the exit site lies in a reasonable location. The patient should be placed head-down to avoid air embolism. In patients with impaired renal function, the subclavian route for dialysis catheters should only be used as a last resort, as there is a 50 % incidence of subclavian vein stenosis. This can lead to problems if a fistula is created in the ipsilateral arm. When using the open approach, a cervical skin crease incision is placed over the carotid pulsation, 1 finger width above the clavicle. The SVC is secured above and below the venotomy site, and the largest catheter for the vein size is inserted. A circumferential 6/0 Prolene suture closes the venotomy against the catheter. Some catheters have a small Dacron cuff, which is positioned under the skin, to fixate the catheter.

Anatomical Points

The position of the subclavian and internal jugular veins is relatively constant; however, there is some relative minor variation, due to differences in the surrounding bony anatomy between individuals and the hydration status of the patient. Dehydration decreases venous size and can make access more difficult. The internal jugular vein can overlie or even be medial to the carotid artery in some patients, and ultrasound guidance may be of value. Placing the patient slightly "head-down" is also helpful in dilating the venous system of the head and neck facilitating easier entry of the initial needle and reducing risk of air embolism. The pleura lies behind the medial 1/3 of the clavicle on each side and is at risk of puncture and inducing a pneumothorax.

Perspective

See Table 6.2. The procedure is usually associated with a low complication rate, and most are minor, such as bruising, difficulty gaining access to the vein, and minor superficial infection. Life-threatening complications are rare and less common than by the subclavian route. Major complications are rare but can occur, such as pneumothorax, which may require further hospitalization or insertion of an underwater-seal chest drain tube. Air embolus is very rare, especially with the

Table 6.2 Tunneled internal jugular line insertion estimated frequency of complications, risks, and consequences

Complications, risks, and consequences	Estimated frequency
Most significant/serious complications	
Infection (overall)[a]	20–50 %
Wound	1–5 %
Related to the catheter	5–20 %
Systemic sepsis	1–5 %
Bleeding/hematoma formation[a]	
Wound	1–5 %
Thrombosis – SVC thrombosis/internal jugular/cephalic vein[a]	1–5 %
Nerve injury (depending on positioning) [cutaneous nerve, Vagus X nerve damage, etc.]	<0.1 %
Catheter failure (from whatever cause) [misdirection, occlusion, kinking, fracture/breakage, too long/short]	1–5 %
Rare significant/serious problems	
Catheter tip embolus	<0.1 %
Air embolism	<0.1 %
Cardiac arrhythmias (catheter irritation of endocardium)	0.1–1 %
Pneumothorax (rare with int. jugular cannulation)[a]	0.1–1 %
Migration/displacement of the catheter tube	0.1–1 %
Catheter or guidewire vascular perforation[a]	<0–1 %
Cardiac perforation and tamponade[a]	<0–1 %
Hemothorax (rare with int. jugular cannulation)	<0–1 %
Thoracic duct injury (left side only)	<0–1 %
Laryngeal edema	<0–1 %
Multisystem organ failure[a]	<0–1 %
Death[a]	<0–1 %
Less serious complications	
Residual pain/discomfort/neuralgia	1–5 %
Wound dehiscence	1–5 %
Skin necrosis	0.1–1 %
Radiation exposure (for the patient) (low level)	>80 %
Bruising	20–50 %
Failure to perform catheter insertion (technical problems) (depends on number of previous catheterizations in dialysis patients and use of U/S)	1–5 %
Seroma/lymphocele/lymphatic leak	1–5 %
Delayed wound healing (including ulceration)	1–5 %
Wound scarring (poor cosmesis)	1–5 %

[a]Dependent on underlying pathology, anatomy, surgical technique, preferences, and comorbidities

"head-down" patient position is used. Cardiac arrhythmias and bleeding are risks during insertion. Immediate withdrawal of the catheter wire or tube several centimeters will usually settle the arrhythmia. Catheter thrombosis, cardiac arrhythmias, and migration of the catheter are also potentially serious as the catheter may require removal and later reinsertion. Percutaneous CVC lines invariably fail over time due to infection, mechanical problems, or thrombosis, and regular replacement may avert these issues as clinical complications. Failure to complete the procedure by the percutaneous method will not usually disallow its insertion, since the open approach can usually be then used. Bilateral attempts at central line insertion via the subclavian approach are not advisable within 24 h of each other, as there is a risk of inducing bilateral pneumothoraces. Use of the internal jugular approach is preferable after a failed subclavian approach or in patients with renal impairment.

Major Complications

The main severe acute complications are **pneumothorax, cardiac arrhythmias, air embolism,** and **hemothorax.** Later, **infection** of the catheter line can lead to **systemic sepsis** and even **multisystem organ failure**, which is the major cause of **mortality**, especially in immunocompromised patients and severely ill patients. **Catheter tip bacterial colonization or thrombosis** with consequent **embolization** of material can occur and may be associated with bacterial endocarditis or metastatic infection. **Removal of the central line** invariably follows infection. Air embolism, pneumothorax, and hemothorax are very rare with the jugular approach, but can be life-threatening. **Catheter blockage or leakage** due to a variety of problems may require removal and reinsertion or adjustment. **Catheter tip migration** can occur into the jugular (or subclavian depending on the vessel of insertion) vein, opposite subclavian vein, right heart, IVC, or even pulmonary artery but is relatively rare as the cuff holds it in place. **Catheter fracture and embolism** is reported and may require radiological or rarely open surgical removal. **Axillary, subclavian, internal jugular, or superior vena cava venous** thrombosis can cause severe swelling of the arm, neck, head, and chest. **Failure to thread the wire** can be a problem, particularly in renal patients who have had previous central venous lines. **Carotid artery puncture** may be minimized by the use of ultrasound guidance. **Cardiac arrhythmias** are common when the guidewire enters the heart chamber, usually irritating the sinoatrial node, usually terminated by withdrawal of the catheter from the right atrium into the SVC. **Catheter or guidewire vascular perforation** is very rare, especially with J-hooked, soft-tipped guidewires or soft catheters, but both are well reported. **Cardiac perforation and tamponade** is exceedingly rare.

Consent and Risk Reduction

Main Points to Explain

- Discomfort
- Bruising and bleeding
- Infection
- Pneumothorax (rare)
- Cardiac arrhythmias (usually minor)
- Failure of insertion
- Catheter displacement/later failure
- Further surgery

Venous Access Devices (Infusion Port) Insertion
Percutaneous Insertion

Description

General anesthesia is usually preferable; however, local anesthesia may be used on occasions. The aim is to gain access to the subclavian or internal jugular vein using a percutaneous Seldinger technique (guidewire, dilator, separable sheath, Silastic catheter). A separate subcutaneous pocket is made for the port, which is attached to the Silastic catheter. The catheter is tunneled to reach the sheath and inserted into the vein, and then the sheath can be stripped away. The position of the catheter in the superior vena cava can then be checked using image intensification radiology. The skin is then closed to render the whole system subcutaneous.

Anatomical Points

The position of the subclavian and internal jugular veins is relatively constant; however, there is some relative variation, due to differences in the surrounding bony anatomy between individuals. Placing the patient slightly "head-down" is also helpful in dilating the venous system of the head and neck facilitating easier entry of the initial needle and reducing air embolism. The pleura lies behind the medial 1/3 of the clavicle on each side and is at risk of puncture and inducing a pneumothorax.

Perspective

See Table 6.3. The procedure is usually associated with a low complication rate and most or minor, such as bruising, difficulty gaining access to the vein, minor superficial infection, and seroma. Major immediate complications are rare but can occur, such as pneumothorax, which may require further hospitalization or insertion of a chest underwater-seal drain tube, or cardiac arrhythmias, which can be serious. Infection, sepsis, and thrombosis are potentially serious later complications and frequently lead to port removal. Leakage from the port, port infection, catheter thrombosis, and migration of the catheter (either operatively or later) are also potentially serious as the port and catheter may require removal and later reinsertion. Failure to complete the procedure by the percutaneous method will not usually disallow its insertion, since the open approach can usually be then used. Port rotation or leakage can prevent use and are technical complications averted with careful 3-point fixation of the port and use of the correct (Huber) needle type, respectively.

Table 6.3 Open venous access devices (including infusion port) insertion estimated frequency of complications, risks, and consequences

Complications, risks, and consequences	Estimated frequency
Most significant/serious complications	
Infection (overall)	1–5 %
Wound	1–5 %
Within the port	1–5 %
Systemic sepsis	0.1–1 %
Bleeding or hematoma formation	
Wound	1–5 %
Bruising	20–50 %
Thrombosis – SVC/internal jugular/SCV/axillary/cephalic vein	1–5 %
Catheter failure (from whatever cause) [misdirection, occlusion, kinking, fracture/breakage, too long/short]	1–5 %
Port leakage/extravasation	1–5 %
Rare significant/serious problems	
Pneumothorax (rare with int. jugular cannulation)[a]	0.1–1 %
Cardiac arrhythmias (catheter irritation of endocardium)	0.1–1 %
Catheter tip embolus	0.1–1 %
Nerve injury (depending on positioning) [cutaneous nerve, Vagus X nerve damage, brachial plexus, etc.]	0.1–1 %
Catheter or guidewire vascular perforation[a]	<0.1 %
Cardiac perforation and tamponade[a]	<0.1 %
Subclavian vein fistula/injury	<0.1 %
Hemothorax	<0.1 %
Air embolism	<0.1 %
Thoracic duct injury (left side)	<0.1 %
Multisystem organ failure[a]	<0.1 %
Death[a]	<0.1 %
Less serious complications	
Seroma/lymphocele/lymphatic leak	1–5 %
Failure to perform port insertion (technical problems)	0.1–1 %
Migration/displacement/rotation of port or catheter tube	1–5 %
Fat necrosis	0.1–1 %
Radiation exposure (for the patient) (low level)	>80 %
Foreign body reaction	1–5 %
Wound dehiscence	1–5 %
Skin necrosis/port erosion	0.1–1 %
Residual pain/discomfort/neuralgia	1–5 %
Delayed wound healing (including ulceration)	1–5 %
Wound scarring (poor cosmesis)	1–5 %

[a]Dependent on underlying pathology, anatomy, surgical technique, and preferences

Major Complications

The main severe acute complications are **pneumothorax, cardiac arrhythmias, air embolism,** and **hemothorax.** Later, **infection** of the catheter line can lead to **systemic sepsis** and even **multisystem organ failure**, which is the major cause of **mortality**, especially in immunocompromised patients and severely ill patients. **Catheter tip bacterial colonization or thrombosis** with consequent **embolization** of material can occur and may be associated with bacterial endocarditis or metastatic infection. **Removal of the port and central line** invariably follows infection. **Port rotation or leakage** can prevent use and may require adjustment or removal. Air embolism, pneumothorax, and hemothorax are very rare with the jugular approach, but can be life-threatening. **Catheter blockage or leakage** due to a variety of problems may require removal and reinsertion or adjustment. **Catheter tip migration** can occur into the jugular (or subclavian depending on the vessel of insertion) vein, opposite subclavian vein, right heart, IVC, or even pulmonary artery but is relatively rare as the cuff holds it in place. **Catheter fracture and embolism** is reported and may require radiological or rarely open surgical removal. **Axillary, subclavian, internal jugular, or superior vena cava venous** thrombosis can cause severe swelling of the arm, neck, head, and chest. **Failure to thread the wire** can be a problem, particularly in renal patients who have had previous central venous lines. **Carotid artery puncture** may be minimized by the use of ultrasound guidance. **Cardiac arrhythmias** are common when the guidewire enters the heart chamber, usually irritating the sinoatrial node, usually terminated by withdrawal of the catheter from the right atrium into the SVC. **Catheter or guidewire vascular perforation** is very rare, especially with J-hooked, soft-tipped guidewires or soft catheters, but both are well reported. **Cardiac perforation and tamponade** is exceedingly rare.

Consent and Risk Reduction

Main Points to Explain

- Discomfort
- Bruising and bleeding
- Infection
- Pneumothorax (rare)
- Cardiac arrhythmias (usually minor)
- Failure of insertion
- Catheter displacement/later failure
- Further surgery

Venous Access Devices (Infusion Port) Insertion
Open Surgical Insertion

Description

General anesthesia is usually preferable; however, local anesthesia may be used on occasions. The aim is to gain access to the subclavian or internal jugular vein using an open surgical technique. A separate subcutaneous pocket is made for the port, which is attached to the Silastic catheter. The catheter is tunneled to the insertion point into the vein and secured using a purse-string suture. The position of the catheter in the superior vena cava can then be checked using image intensification radiology. Occasionally, a Seldinger-type approach can be used with a guidewire, but almost always the catheter is inserted directly into the vein. The skin is then closed to render the whole system subcutaneous. The open approach is most often used when the subclavian percutaneous approach is compromised or inadvisable, for example, due to previous pneumothoraces, multiple previous central venous lines, or local skin problems.

Anatomical Points

The position of the subclavian and internal jugular veins is relatively constant; however, there is some relative variation, due to differences in the surrounding bony anatomy between individuals. Placing the patient slightly "head-down" is also helpful in dilating the venous system of the head and neck facilitating easier entry of the initial needle and reducing air embolism. The pleura lies behind the medial 1/3 of the clavicle on each side and is at risk of puncture and inducing a pneumothorax.

Perspective

See Table 6.4. The procedure is usually associated with a low complication rate and most or minor, such as bruising, difficulty gaining access to the vein, minor superficial infection, and seroma. Major complications are rare but can occur, such as pneumothorax (although much less than for the subclavian percutaneous approach), which may require further hospitalization or insertion of a chest underwater-seal drain tube. Leakage from the port, port infection, catheter thrombosis, cardiac arrhythmias, and migration of the catheter are also potentially serious as the port and catheter may require removal and later reinsertion. Failure to complete the procedure by the open method is very rare. Port rotation and leakage can prevent use and are technical complications averted with careful 3-point fixation of the port and use of the correct (Huber) needle type, respectively.

Major Complications

The main severe acute complications are **cardiac arrhythmias and air embolism. Pneumothorax** and **hemothorax** are very rare using open insertion techniques. Later**, infection** of the catheter line can lead to **systemic sepsis** and even **multisystem organ failure**, which is the major cause of **mortality**, especially in immunocompromised patients and severely ill patients. **Catheter tip bacterial colonization or thrombosis** with consequent **embolization** of material can occur and may be

Table 6.4 Percutaneous venous access devices (including infusion port) insertion estimated frequency of complications, risks, and consequences

Complications, risks, and consequences	Estimated frequency
Most significant/serious complications	
Infection (overall)	1–5 %
Wound	1–5 %
Within the port	1–5 %
Systemic sepsis	0.1–1 %
Bleeding or hematoma formation – wound[a]	1–5 %
Bruising	20–50 %
Thrombosis – SVC/internal jugular/SCV/axillary/cephalic veins	1–5 %
Migration/displacement of the port or catheter tube	1–5 %
Catheter failure (from whatever cause) [misdirection, occlusion, kinking, fracture/breakage, too long/short]	1–5 %
Port leakage/rotation	1–5 %
Rare significant/serious problems	
Cardiac arrhythmias (catheter irritation of endocardium)	0.1–1 %
Nerve injury (depending on positioning) [cutaneous nerve, Vagus X nerve damage, brachial plexus, etc.]	0.1–1 %
Failure to perform port insertion (technical problems)	0.1–1 %
Catheter tip embolus	0.1–1 %
Subclavian vein fistula	<0.1 %
Pneumothorax	<0.1 %
Hemothorax	<0.1 %
Multisystem organ failure[a]	<0.1 %
Death[a]	<0.1 %
Air embolism	<0.1 %
Less serious complications	
Radiation exposure (for the patient) (low level)	>80 %
Residual pain/discomfort/neuralgia	1–5 %
Wound dehiscence	1–5 %
Seroma/lymphocele/lymphatic leak	1–5 %
Foreign body reaction	1–5 %
Skin necrosis	0.1–1 %
Fat necrosis	0.1–1 %
Delayed wound healing (including ulceration)	1–5 %
Wound scarring (poor cosmesis)	1–5 %

[a]Dependent on underlying pathology, anatomy, surgical technique, and preferences

associated with bacterial endocarditis or metastatic infection. **Removal of the port and central line** invariably follows infection. **Port rotation or leakage** can prevent use and may require adjustment or removal. Air embolism, pneumothorax, and hemothorax are very rare with the jugular approach but can be life-threatening. **Catheter blockage or leakage** due to a variety of problems may require removal and reinsertion or adjustment. **Catheter tip migration** can occur into the jugular (or subclavian depending on the vessel of insertion) vein, opposite subclavian vein, right heart, IVC, or even pulmonary artery but is relatively rare as the cuff holds it in place. **Catheter fracture and embolism** is reported and may require radiological or rarely open surgical removal. **Axillary, subclavian, internal jugular, or**

superior vena cava venous thrombosis can cause severe swelling of the arm, neck, head, and chest. **Failure to thread the wire** (where a wire is used) can be a problem, particularly in renal patients who have had previous central venous lines. **Carotid artery puncture** is extremely rare with direct open access. **Cardiac arrhythmias** are common when the guidewire enters the heart chamber, usually irritating the sinoatrial node, usually terminated by withdrawal of the catheter from the right atrium into the SVC. **Catheter or guidewire vascular perforation** is very rare, especially with J-hooked, soft-tipped guidewires or soft catheters, but both are well reported. **Cardiac perforation and tamponade** is exceedingly rare.

Consent and Risk Reduction

Main Points to Explain

- Discomfort
- Bruising and bleeding
- Infection
- Pneumothorax (rare)
- Cardiac arrhythmias (usually minor)
- Failure of insertion
- Catheter displacement/later failure
- Further surgery

Hepatic Arterial Catheter Insertion

Description

General anesthesia is used. The usual indication for this procedure is for longer-term administration of chemotherapeutic agents intra-arterially, often by slow continuous infusion. The catheter can be inserted open laparotomy, occasionally laparoscopically or with increasing frequency angiographically. Prophylactic antibiotics should be given. The catheter is placed into the hepatic artery and secured using a ligature. The catheter tube is first passed through the anterior or lateral abdominal wall to the port, typically located subcutaneously, being secured with stay sutures to the fascia of the abdominal wall musculature. The port can then be accessed using direct transcutaneous puncture through the silicone diaphragm as required.

Anatomical Points

The hepatic artery arises from the coeliac trunk and lies within the free right edge of the lesser omentum, anterior and medial to the portal vein, and the common bile

Table 6.5 Hepatic arterial infusion port insertion estimated frequency of complications, risks, and consequences

Complications, risks, and consequences	Estimated frequency
Most significant/serious complications	
Infection (overall acute and chronic)[a]	5–20 %
Wound	1–5 %
Peritonitis (operation related)	0.1–1 %
Systemic sepsis	0.1–1 %
Bruising	20–50 %
Bleeding or hematoma formation	
Wound	1–5 %
Intra-abdominal	0.1–1 %
Migration/displacement of the catheter tube	5–20 %
Migration/displacement of the catheter tube causing flow problems	1–5 %
Leak	5–20 %
Hernia/prolapse	5–20 %
Catheter failure (from whatever cause)	5–20 %
Peritoneal adhesions	1–5 %
Small bowel obstruction (early or late)	1–5 %
Rare significant/serious problems	
Bowel perforation	0.1–1 %
Bladder perforation[a]	0.1–1 %
Cuff erosion	0.1–1 %
Failure to perform catheter insertion (adhesions)[a]	0.1–1 %
Multisystem organ failure[a]	<0.1 %
Death[a]	<0.1 %
Less serious complications	
Paralytic ileus	1–5 %
Wound dehiscence	1–5 %
Residual pain/discomfort/neuralgia	1–5 %
Skin necrosis	0.1–1 %
Seroma	0.1–1 %
Delayed wound healing (including ulceration)	1–5 %
Wound scarring (poor cosmesis)[a]	1–5 %

[a]Dependent on underlying pathology, anatomy, surgical technique, and preferences

duct as the three structures extend to the porta hepatis. The hepatic artery is relatively constant in position but occasionally can be smaller in caliber than expected, making cannulation difficult.

Perspective

See Table 6.5. Failure of cannulation is possible when a very small caliber vessel is present. Bleeding may occur, and injury to the portal vein or common bile duct is potentially a serious problem. Hematoma formation may lead to infection and rarely abscess formation. Dislodgement of the catheter from vigorous flushing or failure to secure the catheter properly can result in leakage of the infused chemotherapy agent, with potentially serious consequences. A chemical peritonitis or toxicity may occur, depending on the agent, extent of leakage, and quantity leaked. Infusion port problems, including rotation, leakage, infection, blockage, and thrombosis, can occur.

Major Complications

The two most important perioperative complications are **failure of infusion (function)** and **peritoneal leakage** of infused chemotherapy. Testing of the catheter and port intraoperatively and adequately securing the catheter can reduce these risks. **Peritonitis**, either chemical or infective or both, and **wound or systemic infection** are potential serious problems. These may cause significant morbidity and rarely lead to **multisystem organ failure** and potentially early **death**. **Bleeding** and **visceral organ injury** are rare and should be avoidable. **Infusion port problems**, including rotation, leakage, infection, blockage, and thrombosis, can occur.

Consent and Risk Reduction

Main Points to Explain

- Discomfort
- Bruising and bleeding
- Infection
- Pneumothorax (rare)
- Cardiac arrhythmias (usually minor)
- Failure of insertion
- Catheter displacement/later failure
- Further surgery

Peritoneal Dialysis Catheter Insertion

Description

General anesthesia, spinal anesthesia, or local anesthetic and sedation can be used. The catheter can be inserted open or laparoscopically. Prophylactic antibiotics should be given. The catheter is placed behind the bladder, as the dialysis fluid sits in the pelvis and drains out by a siphon effect. The peritoneum is carefully closed, with a "Dacron" cuff external to the peritoneum. The catheter is tunneled to (usually) the left iliac fossa, with the subcutaneous Dacron cuff about 1 cm away from the exit site. The exit site should point downwards to allow drainage of any infection. The catheter can also be placed laparoscopically, taking care to close the portholes.

Anatomical Points

A patent pleuroperitoneal canal can exist, allowing peritoneal dialysis fluid to accumulate in the chest. This can be treated by pleurodesis but not always with success. Adhesions, either congenital or acquired after previous surgery, can limit fluid movement and access to the pelvis during insertion or subsequently with use of the catheter. Reinsertion of peritoneal dialysis catheters may be difficult due to peritoneal adhesions, more commonly induced by repeated infections.

Perspective

See Table 6.6. Failure of peritoneal dialysis is usually due to leaks or drainage problems. Both these usually lead to periods away from peritoneal dialysis (usually on hemodialysis) and often further surgery. Peritoneal adhesions and infections may cause problems with fluid loculations and difficult drainage and/or pain.

Table 6.6 Peritoneal dialysis catheter insertion estimated frequency of complications, risks, and consequences

Complications, risks, and consequences	Estimated frequency
Most significant/serious complications	
Infection (overall acute and chronic)[a]	5–20 %
Wound	1–5 %
Peritonitis (operation related)	0.1–1 %
Systemic sepsis	0.1–1 %
Bruising	20–50 %
Bleeding or hematoma formation	
Wound	1–5 %
Intra-abdominal	0.1–1 %
Migration/displacement of the catheter tube	5–20 %
Migration/displacement of the catheter tube causing flow problems	1–5 %
Leak	5–20 %
Catheter failure (from whatever cause)[b]	5–20 %
Peritoneal adhesions	1–5 %
Small bowel obstruction (early or late)	1–5 %
Rare significant/serious problems	
Bowel perforation[b]	0.1–1 %
Bladder perforation[b]	0.1–1 %
Cuff erosion	0.1–1 %
Failure to perform catheter insertion (adhesions)[b]	0.1–1 %
Multisystem organ failure[a]	<0.1 %
Death[a]	<0.1 %

(continued)

Table 6.6 (continued)

Complications, risks, and consequences	Estimated frequency
Less serious complications	
Residual pain/discomfort/neuralgia	1–5 %
Paralytic ileus	1–5 %
Skin necrosis	0.1–1 %
Seroma	0.1–1 %
Hernia/prolapse	5–20 %
Delayed wound healing (including ulceration)	1–5 %
Wound dehiscence	1–5 %
Wound scarring (poor cosmesis)[a]	1–5 %

[a]Dependent on underlying pathology, anatomy, surgical technique, and preferences
[b]Increased risk with multiple adhesions, recurrent catheter insertions, or without imaging

Major Complications

The two most important perioperative complications are **peritoneal leaks** and **failure of drainage of the catheter**. Leaks can be limited by careful closure of the peritoneum or port sites and allowing a period of at least 2 weeks prior to use. Failure of drainage out is often due to omental wrapping, the fluid flowing in easily as the pressure lifts the omentum away. There may also be adhesions of small bowel around the catheter, causing a similar problem. This usually requires further surgery +/− omentectomy. **Bleeding** and **visceral organ injury** are rare and should be avoidable. A cuff placed too superficially (<1 cm below the skin) can cause **skin erosion** with time. **Infection** is usually limited by the use of perioperative antibiotics but can occur later with a spectrum from **local infection** around the catheter entry site, **cellulitis**, **peritonitis**, **systemic infection,** and rarely **multisystem organ failure**.

Consent and Risk Reduction

Main Points to Explain

- Discomfort
- Bruising and bleeding
- Infection
- Pneumothorax (rare)
- Cardiac arrhythmias (usually minor)
- Failure of insertion
- Catheter displacement/later failure
- Further surgery

Further Reading, References, and Resources

Central Venous Line Insertion

Braner DAV, Lai S, Eman S, Tegtmeyer K. Central venous catheterization—subclavian vein. N Engl J Med. 2007;357:e26.

Clemente CD. Anatomy – a regional atlas of the human body. 4th ed. Baltimore: Williams and Wilkins; 1997.

Fortune JB, Feustel P. Effect of patient position on size and location of the subclavian vein for percutaneous puncture. Arch Surg. 2003;138:996–1000.

Jamieson GG. The anatomy of general surgical operations. 2nd ed. Edinburgh: Churchill Livingston; 2006.

Orihashi K, Imai K, Sato K, Hamamoto M, Okada K, Sueda T. Extrathoracic subclavian venipuncture under ultrasound guidance. Circ J. 2005;69:1111–5.

Pirotte T, Veyckemans F. Ultrasound guided subclavian vein cannulation in infants and children: a novel approach. Br J Anaesth. 2007;98:509–14.

Tunneled Internal Jugular Line Insertion

Clemente CD. Anatomy – a regional atlas of the human body. 4th ed. Baltimore: Williams and Wilkins; 1997.

Conlon PJ, Schwab SJ, Nicholson ML, editors. Hemodialysis vascular access: practice and problems. New York: Oxford University Press; 2000.

Jamieson GG. The anatomy of general surgical operations. 2nd ed. Edinburgh: Churchill Livingston; 2006.

Levy J, Morgan J, Brown E editors. Oxford handbook of dialysis. Chapter in haemodialysis. Oxford: Oxford University Press; 2001.

Lin B, Kong C, Tarng D, Huang T, Tang G. Anatomical variation of the internal jugular vein and its impact on temporary haemodialysis vascular access: an ultrasonographic survey in uraemic patients. Nephrol Dial Transplant. 1998;13:134–8.

Open Venous Access Devices (Including Infusion Port) Insertion

Brothers TE, Von Moll LK, Niederhuber JE, Roberts JA, Walker-Andrews S, Ensminger WD. Experience with subcutaneous infusion ports in three hundred patients. Surg Gynecol Obstet. 1988;166(4):295–301.

Carlo JT, Lamont JP, McCarty TM, Livingston S, Kuhn JA. A prospective randomized trial demonstrating valved implantable ports have fewer complications and lower overall cost than nonvalved implantable ports. Am J Surg. 2004;188(6):722–7.

Clemente CD. Anatomy – a regional atlas of the human body. 4th ed. Baltimore: Williams and Wilkins; 1997.

Eastridge BJ, Lefor AT. Complications of indwelling venous access devices in cancer patients. J Clin Oncol. 1995;13(1):233–8.

Gonsalves CF, Eschelman DJ, Sullivan KL, DuBois N, Bonn J. Incidence of central vein stenosis and occlusion following upper extremity PICC and port placement. Cardiovasc Intervent Radiol. 2003;26(2):123–7.

Jamieson GG. The anatomy of general surgical operations. 2nd ed. Edinburgh: Churchill
    Livingston; 2006.
Lamont JP, McCarty TM, Stephens JS, Smith BA, Carlo J, Livingston S, Kuhn JA. A randomized
    trial of valved vs nonvalved implantable ports for vascular access. Proc (Bayl Univ Med Cent).
    2003;16(4):384–7.
Power Port Implanted Port Device Manual. Salt lake City; Bard Access Systems Inc; 2009.
Raaf JH. Results from use of 826 vascular access devices in cancer patients. Cancer.
    1985;55(6):1312–21.
Seiler CM, Frohlich BE, Dorsam UJ, Kienle P, Buchler MW, Knaebel HP. Surgical technique for
    totally implantable access ports (TIAP) needs improvement: a multivariate analysis of 400
    patients. J Surg Oncol. 2006;93(1):24–9.
Soh LT, Ang PT. Implantable subcutaneous infusion ports. Support Care Cancer. 1993;1(2):108–10.
Viale PH. Complications associated with implantable vascular access devices in the patient with
    cancer. J Infus Nurs. 2003;26(2):97–102. Review.

Percutaneous Venous Access Devices (Including Infusion Port) Insertion

Brothers TE, Von Moll LK, Niederhuber JE, Roberts JA, Walker-Andrews S, Ensminger WD.
    Experience with subcutaneous infusion ports in three hundred patients. Surg Gynecol Obstet.
    1988;166(4):295–301.
Carlo JT, Lamont JP, McCarty TM, Livingston S, Kuhn JA. A prospective randomized trial
    demonstrating valved implantable ports have fewer complications and lower overall cost than
    nonvalved implantable ports. Am J Surg. 2004;188(6):722–7.
Clemente CD. Anatomy – a regional atlas of the human body. 4th ed. Baltimore: Williams and
    Wilkins; 1997.
Eastridge BJ, Lefor AT. Complications of indwelling venous access devices in cancer patients.
    J Clin Oncol. 1995;13(1):233–8.
Gonsalves CF, Eschelman DJ, Sullivan KL, DuBois N, Bonn J. Incidence of central vein stenosis
    and occlusion following upper extremity PICC and port placement. Cardiovasc Intervent
    Radiol. 2003;26(2):123–7.
Jamieson GG. The anatomy of general surgical operations. 2nd ed. Edinburgh: Churchill
    Livingston; 2006.
Lamont JP, McCarty TM, Stephens JS, Smith BA, Carlo J, Livingston S, Kuhn JA. A randomized
    trial of valved vs nonvalved implantable ports for vascular access. Proc (Bayl Univ Med Cent).
    2003;16(4):384–7.
Raaf JH. Results from use of 826 vascular access devices in cancer patients. Cancer.
    1985;55(6):1312–21.
Seiler CM, Frohlich BE, Dorsam UJ, Kienle P, Buchler MW, Knaebel HP. Surgical technique for
    totally implantable access ports (TIAP) needs improvement: a multivariate analysis of 400
    patients. J Surg Oncol. 2006;93(1):24–9.
Soh LT, Ang PT. Implantable subcutaneous infusion ports. Support Care Cancer. 1993;1(2):108–10.
Viale PH. Complications associated with implantable vascular access devices in the patient with
    cancer. J Infus Nurs. 2003;26(2):97–102. Review.

Hepatic Arterial Infusion Port Insertion

Allen PJ, Nissan A, Picon AI, Kemeny N, Dudrick P, Ben-Porat L, Espat J, Stojadinovic A, Cohen
    AM, Fong Y, Paty PB. Technical complications and durability of hepatic artery infusion pumps
    for unresectable colorectal liver metastases: an institutional experience of 544 consecutive
    cases. J Am Coll Surg. 2005;201(1):57–65.

Arai Y, Takeuchi Y, Inaba Y, Yamaura H, Sato Y, Aramaki T, Matsueda K, Seki H. Percutaneous catheter placement for hepatic arterial infusion chemotherapy. Tech Vasc Interv Radiol. 2007;10(1):30–7. Review.

Clemente CD. Anatomy – a regional atlas of the human body. 4th ed. Baltimore: Williams and Wilkins; 1997.

Franklin M, Trevino J, Hernandez-Oaknin H, Fisher T, Berghoff K. Laparoscopic hepatic artery catheterization for regional chemotherapy: is this the best current option for liver metastatic disease? Surg Endosc. 2006;20(4):554–8.

Ganeshan A, Upponi S, Hon LQ, Warakaulle D, Uberoi R. Hepatic arterial infusion of chemotherapy: the role of diagnostic and interventional radiology. Ann Oncol. 2008;19(5): 847–51.

Hellan M, Pigazzi A. Robotic-assisted placement of a hepatic artery infusion catheter for regional chemotherapy. Surg Endosc. 2008;22(2):548–51.

Jamieson GG. The anatomy of general surgical operations. 2nd ed. Edinburgh: Churchill Livingston; 2006.

Noda T, Ohigashi H, Ishikawa O, Eguchi H, Yamada T, Sasaki Y, Yano M, Imaoka S. Liver perfusion chemotherapy for selected patients at a high-risk of liver metastasis after resection of duodenal and ampullary cancers. Ann Surg. 2007;246(5):799–805.

Oberfield RA, Sampson E, Heatley GJ. Hepatic artery infusion chemotherapy for metastatic colorectal cancer to the liver at the Lahey clinic: comparison between two methods of treatment, surgical versus percutaneous catheter placement. Am J Clin Oncol. 2004;27(4): 376–83.

Osborne D, Pappas E, Alexander G, Boe B, Cantor AB, Rosemurgy A, Zervos E. A complication-free course ensures a survival advantage in patients after regional therapy for metastatic colorectal cancer. Am Surg. 2006;72(6):505–10.

Ricke J, Hildebrandt B, Miersch A, Nicolaou A, Warschewske G, Teichgräber U, Lopez Hänninen E, Riess H, Felix R. Hepatic arterial port systems for treatment of liver metastases: factors affecting patency and adverse events. J Vasc Interv Radiol. 2004;15(8):825–33.

Seki H, Ozaki T, Shiina M. Side-hole catheter placement for hepatic arterial infusion chemotherapy in patients with liver metastases from colorectal cancer: long-term treatment and survival benefit. AJR Am J Roentgenol. 2008;190(1):111–20.

Van Nieuwenhove Y, Aerts M, Neyns B, Delvaux G. Techniques for the placement of hepatic artery catheters for regional chemotherapy in unresectable liver metastases. Eur J Surg Oncol. 2007; 33(3):336–40.

Watanabe M, Yamazaki K, Yajima S, Tsuchiya M, Ito M, Nanami T, Oshima Y, Kaneko H, Shimokawa K. Introducing the coaxial method of catheter port implantation for hepatic arterial infusion chemotherapy. J Surg Oncol. 2009;99(6):382–5.

Peritoneal Dialysis Catheter Insertion

Clemente CD. Anatomy – a regional atlas of the human body. 4th ed. Baltimore: Williams and Wilkins; 1997.

Jamieson GG. The anatomy of general surgical operations. 2nd ed. Edinburgh: Churchill Livingston; 2006.

Levy J, Morgan J, Brown E. editors. Peritoneal dialysis – chapter in Oxford handbook of dialysis. Oxford: Oxford University Press; 2001.

Nicholson ML, White S. Access for renal replacement therapy In: Morris PJ, editor. Kidney transplantation: principles and practices. 5th ed. Philadelphia: W.B. Saunders; 2001.

Chapter 7
Lung Surgery

Craig Jurisevic, Jayme Bennetts, and Brendon J. Coventry

General Perspective and Overview

The relative risks and complications increase proportionately according to the site, size, and type and complexity of the problem being addressed within the chest and in relation to the age of the patient and other comorbidities. This is principally related to the surgical accessibility, ability to resect, risk of lung injury and respiratory compromise, functional reserve, technical ease, and the ability to achieve correction of the problem.

The main serious complications are **bleeding and infection,** which can be minimized by the adequate exposure, mobilization, technical care, and avoiding lung injury and hematoma formation. Infection is the main sequel of tissue injury, respiratory obstruction, and hematoma formation and may arise from preexisting infection or be newly acquired. This can lead to **pleural infection, lung consolidation, abscess formation,** and **systemic sepsis. Multisystem failure** and **death** remain serious potential complications from thoracic surgery and systemic infection.

Neural injuries are not infrequent potential problems associated with thoracic surgery and access, because intercostal nerves travel beneath each rib and may be involved in direct incision, compression from retractors, or scar formation.

Positioning on the operating table has been associated with increased risk of **deep venous thrombosis** and **nerve palsies,** especially in prolonged procedures. **Limb ischemia, compartment syndrome,** and **ulnar** and **common peroneal**

C. Jurisevic, MD (✉)
Department of Surgery, Royal Adelaide Hospital, Adelaide, Australia
e-mail: jurisevic@ozemail.com.au

J. Bennetts, BMBS, FRACS, FCSANZ
Cardiac and Thoracic Surgery, Flinders Medical Centre, Adelaide, Australia

B.J. Coventry, BMBS, PhD, FRACS, FACS, FRSM
Discipline of Surgery, Royal Adelaide Hospital, University of Adelaide,
L5 Eleanor Harrald Building, North Terrace, 5000 Adelaide, SA, Australia
e-mail: brendon.coventry@adelaide.edu.au

B.J. Coventry (ed.), *Cardio-Thoracic, Vascular, Renal and Transplant Surgery,*
Surgery: Complications, Risks and Consequences,
DOI 10.1007/978-1-4471-5418-1_7, © Springer-Verlag London 2014

nerve palsy are recognized potential complications, which should be checked for, as the patient's position may change during surgery.

Mortality associated with most thoracic surgery procedures is usually low and principally associated with pulmonary infarction or thromboembolism. Procedures involving the pulmonary vessels, vena cava, or larger arteries carry higher risks associated with possible serious bleeding and infection, including increased risk of mortality. Rare failure of stapling devices can cause catastrophic bleeding.

This chapter therefore attempts to draw together in one place, the estimated overall frequencies of the complications associated with thoracic procedures, based on information obtained from the literature and experience. Not all patients are at risk of the full range of listed complications. It must be individualized for each patient and their disease process but represents a guide and summary of the attendant risks, complications, and consequences.

With these factors and facts in mind, the information given in this chapter must be appropriately and discernibly interpreted and used.

Important Note

It should be emphasized that the risks and frequencies that are given here *represent derived figures*. These *figures are best estimates of relative frequencies across most institutions*, not merely the highest-performing ones, and as such are often representative of a number of studies, which include different patients with differing comorbidities and different surgeons. In addition, the risks of complications in lower- or higher-risk patients may lie outside these estimated ranges, and individual clinical judgement is required as to the expected risks communicated to the patient, staff, or for other purposes. The range of risks is also derived from experience and the literature; while risks outside this range may exist, certain risks may be reduced or absent due to variations of procedures or surgical approaches. It is recognized that different patients, practitioners, institutions, regions, and countries may vary in their requirements and recommendations.

For complications related to other associated/additional surgery that may arise during thoracic surgery, see Volume 4 Oesophageal Surgery or Chap. 8 Cardiac Surgery or the relevant volume and chapter.

Bronchoscopy

Description

General anesthesia is usually used, although sedation and local anesthesia can be used for flexible bronchoscopy. As indicated, the bronchoscope used may be rigid or flexible, and both contain a light source for visualization of the area at the end of the scope.

Bronchoscopy is typically a diagnostic, minimally invasive procedure for delineation of endobronchial conditions but may be used to remove foreign material or aspirate secretions, pus, or lavage the bronchial tree. It may be used just prior to thoracic surgery or separately. It involves careful extension of the cervical spine and negotiation of the teeth, tongue, and lips to avoid injury to any of these structures. Bronchoscopy can reach and visualize the region of the second-order bronchi. Biopsies, brushings, and washings can be retrieved for diagnostic purposes.

Anatomical Points

The oral cavity, pharynx, larynx, trachea, main bronchi, and second-order bronchi are relatively constant in anatomical arrangement, varying mainly in size and minor orientation, except when pathology causes distortion.

Perspective

See Table 7.1. Bronchoscopy is a common place, and even outpatient-type procedure, depending on clinician preference, the indication, patient, nature of the problem being investigated and procedure being conducted. It is relatively safe with a low complication rate if conducted with adequate monitoring, care, and skill. A significant number (flexible) bronchoscopies are performed by thoracic diagnostic physicians and also prior to intrathoracic surgical procedures (either rigid or flexible). The main complications are injury to the lips, teeth, throat, larynx, and

Table 7.1 Bronchoscopy estimated frequency of complications, risks, and consequences

Complications, risks, and consequences	Estimated frequency
Most significant/serious complications	
Infection[a]	
Intrathoracic (pneumonia, pleural)	1–5 %
Mediastinitis	0.1–1 %
Systemic	0.1–1 %
Rare significant/serious problems	
Pneumothorax[a]	0.1–1 %
Bleeding/hematoma formation	0.1–1 %
Aspiration pneumonitis[a]	0.1–1 %
Cardiac arrhythmias	0.1–1 %
Venous thrombosis	0.1–1 %
Multisystem organ failure (renal, pulmonary, cardiac failure)[a]	0.1–1 %
Death[a]	<0.1 %
Less serious complications	
Oral injury[a]	0.1–1 %
Surgical emphysema[a]	<0.1 %

[a]Dependent on underlying anatomy, pathology, location of disease, and/or surgical preference

bronchi, all of which are usually minor but on occasions may be major and can even be a source of litigation. Serious complications are relatively rare, but bronchial perforation, pneumothorax, bleeding, and infection can occur.

Major Complications

The most serious complications of bronchoscopy are bronchial **perforation, bleeding,** and **injury to teeth**. This can usually be reduced by careful measures to protect the structures from injury. Bleeding may result from biopsies, especially in patients with coagulation problems. Rarely, **bronchial injury** can result in air leakage and if severe can lead to **surgical emphysema**, pneumomediastinum, mediastinal leakage, and very rarely **infection** or **pneumothorax**. Occasionally **lung infection** may result from lung collapse, mucus plugging, or obstruction due to foreign material. **Aspiration pneumonitis** may occur as the airway is unprotected. **Multisystem organ failure** and **death** are rare, but the incidence is most related to the underlying lung pathology and other comorbidities.

Consent and Risk Reduction

Main Points to Explain

- Discomfort
- Oral/teeth/neck injury
- Airway injury
- Pneumonia
- Pneumothorax (rare)
- Cardiac arrhythmias (usually minor)
- Further surgery

Thoracoscopy

Description

General anesthesia is used. Video-assisted thoracoscopy is a minimally invasive approach to intrathoracic surgical conditions. It involves the formation of several (usually 2–3) thoracoscopy ports. This involves creating 0.5–1-cm skin incisions, with dissection through the intercostal spaces and, thus, into the pleural space. The exact location of these thoracoscopy ports is dictated by the intrathoracic problem in question. For pulmonary parenchymal resections (e.g., lung biopsies), two 1-cm ports are made in the 5th intercostal space, the first in the anterior axillary line and the second in the midaxillary line. A further 5-mm port is made in the 4th intercostal space in the posterior axillary line. These port placements can also be used for resection of anterior mediastinal lesions such as germ cell tumors or thymic masses. To approach the posterior mediastinum, the ports must be made in the 3rd, 4th, and 6th intercostal spaces in a vertical line in a position between the mid and anterior axillary lines. Pleural conditions requiring resection or biopsy (e.g., for the management of malignant pleural effusions) can be approached simply by two ports in the 6th or 7th intercostal space between the mid and anterior axillary lines. These ports are placed in a lower intercostal space than for pulmonary or mediastinal lesions, such that drains can be placed in a more dependent position to allow more complete drainage of pleural fluid (e.g., to allow for an effective pleurodesis in malignant effusions).

Anatomical Points

The abovementioned thoracoscopy sites may have to be varied depending on the position of the lesion to be resected or biopsy to be taken. In particular, lower lobe pulmonary parenchymal lesions often necessitate the use of ports placed in the 6th or 7th intercostal spaces. Pleural adhesions are not uncommon and may prevent successful thoracoscopic surgery. If the pleural space is obliterated, then thoracoscopy will be impossible and the surgeon would need to resort to open thoracotomy. With a partially obliterated pleural space, pleural adhesions can be dissected and allow enough mobilization of the lung to permit the procedure to be carried out thoracoscopically.

Perspective

See Table 7.2. A significant number of intrathoracic surgical procedures are now performed using the thoracoscopic approach. The main limitation of the thoracoscopic approach involves the fact that, by virtue of the inability to palpate intrathoracic organs, small pulmonary parenchymal lesions not evident on visual inspection of the lung alone, may be difficult to locate and thus resect. Serious complications are relatively rare.

Major Complications

The most serious complication of the thoracoscopic approach to intrathoracic pathology is **bleeding** from the intercostal vessels. This can usually be controlled through the thoracoscopy port but rarely will require a **minithoracotomy** (in the same intercostal space) to control the bleeding. **Intercostal neuralgia** can occur

Table 7.2 Thoracoscopy estimated frequency of complications, risks, and consequences

Complications, risks, and consequences	Estimated frequency
Most significant/serious complications	
Infection	
Subcutaneous/wound	1–5 %
Intrathoracic (pneumonia, pleural)	1–5 %
Mediastinitis	0.1–1 %
Systemic	0.1–1 %
Pneumothorax (residual)	1–5 %
Rare significant/serious problems	
Bleeding/hematoma formation	
Wound	0.1–1 %
Hemothorax	0.1–1 %
Pulmonary contusion	0.1–1 %
Surgical emphysema	0.1–1 %
Persistent air leak	0.1–1 %
Pulmonary empyema	0.1–1 %
Pulmonary abscess	0.1–1 %
Recurrent laryngeal nerve injury	0.1–1 %
Bronchopleural fistula	0.1–1 %
Arrhythmias	0.1–1 %
Pericardial effusion	0.1–1 %
Myocardial injury, cardiac failure, MI (hypotension)	0.1–1 %
Pulmonary injury (direct or inferior pulmonary vein injury)	0.1–1 %
Venous thrombosis	0.1–1 %
Diaphragmatic injury paresis (including phrenic nerve injury)[a]	<0.1 %
Diaphragmatic hernia	<0.1 %
Thoracic duct injury (chylous leak, fistula)	<0.1 %
Osteomyelitis of ribs[a]	<0.1 %
Multisystem failure (renal, pulmonary, cardiac failure)[a]	0.1–1 %
Death[a]	<0.1 %
Less serious complications	
Acute wound pain (<4 weeks)	50–80 %
Chronic wound pain (>12 weeks)	0.1–2 %
Wound scarring or port site or minithoracotomy	1–5 %
Deformity of rib or skin (poor cosmesis)	1–5 %

[a]Dependent on underlying anatomy, pathology, location of disease, and/or surgical preference

following thoracoscopy but is significantly less frequent than following open thoracotomy. Inadvertent **injury to the lung** is also possible especially in the presence of dense pleural adhesions, and occasionally, **pneumothorax** or **persistent air leak** may result. Complications specific to the underlying problem and reason for the thoracoscopy may occur. **Basal atelectasis** and sometimes secondary **lung infection** are not uncommon and may affect either lung. **Empyema** and **abscess formation** are very rare but are severe if they occur leading to prolonged hospital stay and other sequelae. **Multisystem organ failure** is extremely serious, the incidence being most related to the underlying lung pathology and other comorbidities.

Consent and Risk Reduction

Main Points to Explain

- Discomfort
- Bruising and bleeding
- Infection
- Persistent pneumothorax (rare)
- Cardiac arrhythmias (usually minor)
- Failure of insertion/resection
- Further surgery

Thoracotomy (Lateral Intercostal or Median Sternotomy)

Description

General anesthesia is used. A thoracotomy can be anterolateral, lateral, posterolateral, full, or manubriosternal depending on the intrathoracic pathology being attended to. Lateral thoracotomy involves a full-thickness incision into the pleural space by way of the intercostal space, with or without removal of rib(s). Thoracotomy alone is typically used for exploration, diagnosis, biopsy, decortication, pleurodesis, and the like.

An *anterolateral thoracotomy* involves an incision between the midclavicular line and the anterior axillary line, usually through the 5th intercostal space.

A true *lateral thoracotomy* involves an incision situated between the anterior and posterior axillary lines usually in the 5th or 6th intercostal space, incising through serratus anterior and the anterior border of the latissimus dorsi muscles. A *full lateral thoracotomy* extends around the chest through the entire intercostal space.

A *posterolateral thoracotomy* involves extension of the lateral thoracotomy skin incision below the tip of the scapula and extending posterosuperiorly between the medial border of the scapula and the vertebral spinous processes. The incision extends through serratus anterior muscle and latissimus dorsi and can also extend to involve the trapezius and paraspinal group of muscles.

An *anterior thoracotomy* involves an incision extending from the parasternal intercostal space to the midaxillary line, usually in the fifth intercostal space. It requires dissection through the serratus anterior muscle and the intercostal muscles.

Once the intercostal muscles and parietal pleura have been dissected, then a retractor is placed between the ribs and opened. To facilitate the opening of the intercostal space (particularly in the older patient with osteoarthritic costovertebral and costochondral joints), a short segment of the posterior rib (either above or below) can be resected. This increases the thoracotomy opening and reduces the incidence of rib fractures and intercostal nerve traction injury in spaces above and below.

A *median sternotomy* involves a skin incision located between the suprasternal notch and the xiphisternum. A midline division of the manubrium, sternal body, and xiphisternal process is then performed, using a bone saw. This incision allows access to the pericardium and medial aspect of both pleural spaces.

Anatomical Points

There are few anatomical variants that affect this procedure; however, chest wall deformities such as pectus excavatum and scoliosis may alter the ease of approach and therefore the complications. Acquired anatomical changes due to disease, including trauma or previous surgery, can also affect the ease and results of surgery. The intercostal nerves are applied closely to the undersides of each rib and are vulnerable to direct trauma or traction trauma during spreading of the ribs.

Perspective

See Table 7.3. The various thoracotomy incisions require significant muscle dissection and result in trauma to the ribs and costovertebral, costotransverse, costochondral, and sterno-chondral joints. Most significant, however, is traction injury to the intercostal nerves as a direct result of rib retraction/spreading/fracture. Thus, postoperative pain is a significant issue. Furthermore, dissection of the parietal pleura, and the introduction of air and blood into the pleural space, results in a pleuritic response, which contributes significantly to the patient's overall pain. Postoperative analgesia in the thoracotomy patient is significantly improved with the use of thoracic epidural catheters and paravertebral (extrapleural) catheters through which analgesia can be administered.

Major Complications

The major complication directly related to a thoracotomy approach is **bleeding**, either from the chest wall musculature or the intercostal vessels. **Intercostal neuralgia**, secondary to intercostal nerve injury and/or scarring, occurs more frequently than in thoracoscopic procedures and can be permanent in a significant number of cases. **Costochondritis** can occur secondary to trauma at the costochondral joints. This may occur not only in the intercostal space involved but also in costochondral joints several ribs above and below the incisions. Inadvertent **injury to the lung** is also possible especially in the presence of dense pleural adhesions, and occasionally, **pneumothorax** or **persistent air leak** may result. Persistent air leak is more common with underlying lung parenchymal disease, particularly COPD. Complications specific to the underlying problem and reason for the thoracotomy may occur. **Basal atelectasis** and sometimes secondary **lung infection** are not uncommon and may

Table 7.3 Thoracotomy estimated frequency of complications, risks, and consequences

Complications, risks, and consequences	Estimated frequency
Most significant/serious complications	
Infection	
Subcutaneous/wound	1–5 %
Intrathoracic (pneumonia, pleural)	1–5 %
Mediastinitis	0.1–1 %
Systemic	0.1–1 %
Persistent pneumothorax	1–5 %
For malignancy	
Unresectability of malignancy/involved resection margins[a]	1–5 %
Recurrence/progressive disease[a]	1–5 %
Rare significant/serious problems	
Pulmonary abscess/empyema	0.1–1 %
Bleeding/hematoma formation (wound/hemothorax/pulmonary contusion)	0.1–1 %
Recurrent laryngeal nerve injury	0.1–1 %
Persistent air leak	0.1–1 %
Bronchopleural fistula	0.1–1 %
Arrhythmias	0.1–1 %
Pericardial effusion	0.1–1 %
Myocardial injury, cardiac failure, MI (hypotension)	0.1–1 %
Pulmonary injury (direct or inferior pulmonary vein injury)	0.1–1 %
Diaphragmatic injury paresis	<0.1 %
Thoracic duct injury (chylous leak, fistula)	<0.1 %
Venous thrombosis +/− pulmonary embolism	0.1–1 %
Multisystem organ failure (renal, pulmonary, cardiac failure)[a]	0.1–1 %
Death[a]	<0.1 %
Including surgery through the diaphragm	
Liver injury/bowel injury/pancreatitis	0.1–1 %
Splenic injury	0.1–1 %
Conservation (consequent limitation to activity; late rupture)	0.1–1 %
Splenectomy	0.1–1 %
Diaphragmatic hernia	<0.1 %
Less serious complications	
Acute wound pain (<4 weeks)	>80 %
Chronic wound pain (>12 weeks)	
Median sternotomy pain	1–5 %
Thoracotomy (chronic intercostal neuralgia/chronic pain syndrome)	20–50 %
Osteomyelitis of ribs[a]	<0.1 %
Sternal wire protrusion/erosion/pain (median sternotomy if used)[a]	0.1–1 %
Surgical emphysema	0.1–1 %
Wound scarring	1–5 %
Deformity of rib/chest or skin (poor cosmesis)	1–5 %
Pleural drain tube(s)[a]	50–80 %

Note: When a thoracotomy includes esophageal or paraesophageal or esophagogastric surgery, it is associated with the risks, consequences, and complications of those additional procedures, and when a thoracotomy is combined with a laparotomy (thoracolaparotomy), the risks, consequences, and complications of laparotomy should also be included

[a]Dependent on underlying pathology, location of disease, and/or surgical preference

affect either lung. **Empyema** and **abscess formation** are very rare but are severe if they occur leading to prolonged hospital stay and other sequelae. **Multisystem organ failure** is extremely serious, the incidence being most related to the underlying lung pathology and other comorbidities, and is associated with **mortality** when it occurs.

Consent and Risk Reduction

Main Points to Explain

- Discomfort/pain
- Bruising and bleeding
- Infection
- Persistent pneumothorax (rare)
- Cardiac arrhythmias (usually minor)
- Failure of access
- Further surgery
- MSOF and death

Partial Lung Resection

Description

General anesthesia is used. A partial lung resection may take the form of a wedge resection, segmental resection, single lobectomy, or bi-lobectomy, greatly facilitated by the use of lung stapling devices. A *wedge resection* involves a non-anatomical resection of a portion of the lung, most commonly for resection of peripheral lung nodules, where the lesion of interest is resected with a small amount of surrounding lung tissue in the shape of a wedge. A *segmental resection* (or segmentectomy) involves resection of the anatomical segment including segmental bronchus arteries and veins and segmental lymph nodes. A *lobectomy* is an anatomical resection of the entire lobe, which includes the lobar pulmonary arterial and venous supply and accompanying lobar lymph nodes. The interlobar fissures (oblique and horizontal on the right and oblique on the left) are commonly incomplete. The fissures can be completed using standard pulmonary stapling devices.

Anatomical Points

Chest wall deformities such as pectus excavatum and scoliosis may alter the ease of approach and therefore the complications. Acquired anatomical changes due to disease, including trauma or previous surgery, can also affect the ease and results of surgery. Fusion of some of the lung fissures may occur making the dissection more difficult. The most common *pulmonary vascular* variation involves the pulmonary venous supply. In 10 % of patients the right middle lobe pulmonary vein drains directly into the inferior pulmonary vein rather than the superior pulmonary vein. In 2–5 % of patients, there may be a single pulmonary vein receiving tributaries from all lobes. The lobar pulmonary arterial and venous supply is very variable, thus necessitating careful dissection and identification of individual lobar and segmental vessels prior to ligation and transection. Anatomical variation of the *bronchial tree* is much less common than that of vascular supply. The intra- and extra-pericardial course of the pulmonary vessels is quite variable, often necessitating the opening of the pericardium for full assessment. This maneuver often allows the surgeon to fully assess the extent of involvement of the vessels by lesions occurring in a central (hilar, mediastinal) location.

Perspective

See Table 7.4. The major debility resulting from partial lung resections (wedge resection, segmentectomy, or lobectomy) is **empyema** (pleural space infection). This occurs more commonly when, after resection, there is a significant residual air space. The other major debility resulting from partial lung resection is post-resection **bronchopleural fistula**. This occurs more commonly in patients with severe underlying lung disease and can result from a leaking bronchial stump or leakage from a pulmonary parenchymal staple line.

Table 7.4 Partial lung resection estimated frequency of complications, risks, and consequences

Complications, risks, and consequences	Estimated frequency
Most significant/serious complications	
Infection	
Subcutaneous/wound	1–5 %
Intrathoracic (pneumonia, pleural)	1–5 %
Mediastinitis	0.1–1 %
Systemic	0.1–1 %
Persistent pneumothorax[a]	1–5 %
Rib resection[a]	20–50 %
Osteomyelitis of ribs[a]	<0.1 %
For malignancy	
Unresectability of malignancy/involved resection margins[a]	1–5 %
Recurrence/progressive disease[a]	1–5 %
Rare significant/serious problems	
Pulmonary abscess/empyema	0.1–1 %
Bleeding/hematoma formation	
Wound	0.1–1 %
Hemothorax	0.1–1 %
Pulmonary contusion	0.1–1 %
Recurrent laryngeal nerve injury	<0.1 %
Persistent air leak[a]	0.1–1 %
Bronchopleural fistula[a]	0.1–1 %
Arrhythmias	0.1–1 %
Pericardial effusion	0.1–1 %

(continued)

Table 7.4 (continued)

Complications, risks, and consequences	Estimated frequency
Myocardial injury, cardiac failure, MI (hypotension)	0.1–1 %
Pulmonary injury (direct or inferior pulmonary vein injury)	0.1–1 %
Venous thrombosis +/– pulmonary embolism	0.1–1 %
Diaphragmatic injury paresis	<0.1 %
Thoracic duct injury (chylous leak, fistula)[a]	<0.1 %
Multisystem organ failure (renal, pulmonary, cardiac failure)[a]	0.1–1 %
Death[a]	<0.1 %
Less serious complications	
Surgical emphysema	0.1–1 %
Deformity of rib/chest or skin (poor cosmesis)	1–5 %

[a]Dependent on underlying pathology, location of disease, and/or surgical preference

Chylothorax can result from damage to the thoracic duct within the chest and occurs more commonly where there has been extensive mediastinal dissection, for example, during a mediastinal lymph node clearance for bronchogenic carcinoma or esophageal resection.

Major Complications

The most serious complications are **empyema** and **abscess formation**. Many patients will require a surgical drainage procedure, with the consequential debility this entails including prolonged hospital stay and other sequelae. Inadvertent **injury to the lung** is also possible especially in the presence of dense pleural adhesions, and occasionally, **pneumothorax** or **persistent air leak** may result. Complications specific to the underlying problem and reason for the partial lung resection may occur. **Basal atelectasis** and sometimes secondary **lung infection** are not uncommon and may affect either lung. **Chylothorax** and **bronchopleural fistula** formation are chronic debilitating problems that delay recovery significantly. **Multisystem organ failure** is extremely serious, the incidence being most related to the underlying lung pathology and other comorbidities and is associated with **mortality** when it occurs.

Consent and Risk Reduction

Main Points to Explain

- Discomfort/pain
- Bruising and bleeding
- Infection
- Persistent pneumothorax (rare)
- Cardiac arrhythmias (usually minor)
- Failure of access/resection
- Further surgery
- MSOF and death

Total Pneumonectomy

Description

General anesthesia is used. A pneumonectomy is performed via a posterolateral thoracotomy. This procedure involves complete mobilization and isolation of the right or left pulmonary arteries and the superior and inferior pulmonary veins. It is occasionally safer to divide the superior pulmonary vein prior to the artery as this may provide better access to the main pulmonary artery. The main stem bronchus is then divided as close to the carina as possible, and the bronchial stump may be buttressed with either a flap of pleura, an intercostal muscle flap, or a pedicled serratus anterior muscle flap. When a pneumonectomy is performed for bronchogenic carcinoma, mediastinal lymph node sampling is a standard part of the procedure.

Anatomical Points

Chest wall deformities such as pectus excavatum and scoliosis may alter the ease of approach and therefore the complications. Acquired anatomical changes due to disease, including trauma or previous surgery, can also affect the ease and results of surgery. Fusion of some of the lung fissures may occur making the dissection more difficult. The most common *pulmonary vascular* variation involves the pulmonary venous supply. In 10 % of patients, the right middle lobe pulmonary vein drains directly into the inferior pulmonary vein rather than the superior pulmonary vein. In 2–5 % of patients, there may be a single pulmonary vein receiving tributaries from all lobes. The lobar pulmonary arterial and venous supply is very variable, thus necessitating careful dissection and identification of individual lobar and segmental vessels prior to ligation and transection. Anatomical variation of the *bronchial tree* is much less common than that of vascular supply. The intra- and extra-pericardial course of the pulmonary vessels is quite variable, often necessitating the opening of the pericardium for full assessment. This maneuver often allows the surgeon to fully assess the extent of involvement of the vessels by lesions occurring in a central (hilar, mediastinal) location.

Perspective

See Table 7.5. Pleural space infection (**empyema**) is more common following pneumonectomy than partial lung resection. This is by virtue of the fact that there is a large residual air space. Fluid eventually fills the cavity. **Bronchopleural fistula** is also a significant problem and occurs more commonly on the right than left due to the more exposed nature of the right main bronchus following pneumonectomy. The incidence of a bronchopleural fistula can be reduced by covering the bronchial stump with a pleural, intercostal muscle flap, or a pedicled serratus anterior flap at

Table 7.5 Total pneumonectomy estimated frequency of complications, risks, and consequences

Complications, risks, and consequences	Estimated frequency
Most significant/serious complications	
Infection[a]	
Subcutaneous/wound	1–5 %
Intrathoracic (pneumonia, pleural)	1–5 %
Mediastinitis	0.1–1 %
Systemic	0.1–1 %
Arrthymias	20–50 %
Persistent pneumothorax[a]	1–5 %
Pulmonary failure[a]	1–5 %
Prolonged assisted ventilation[a]	1–5 %
Multisystem organ failure (renal, pulmonary, cardiac failure)[a]	1–5 %
Death[a]	1–5 %
Right pneumonectomy	1–5 %
Left pneumonectomy	1–2 %
Rare significant/serious problems	
Pulmonary abscess/empyema	0.1–1 %
Bleeding/hematoma formation	
Wound	0.1–1 %
Hemothorax	0.1–1 %
Pulmonary contusion	0.1–1 %
Recurrent laryngeal nerve injury	0.1–1 %
Persistent air leak[a]	0.1–1 %
Bronchopleural fistula[a]	0.1–1 %
Pericardial effusion	0.1–1 %
Myocardial injury, cardiac failure, MI (hypotension)	0.1–1 %
Pulmonary injury (direct or inferior pulmonary vein injury)	0.1–1 %
Esophageal injury[a]	0.1–1 %
Venous thrombosis +/− pulmonary embolism	0.1–1 %
Osteomyelitis of ribs[a]	<0.1 %
Diaphragmatic injury paresis	<0.1 %
Thoracic duct injury (chylous leak, fistula)[a]	<0.1 %
Less serious complications	
Surgical emphysema	0.1–1 %
Deformity of rib/chest or skin (poor cosmesis)	1–5 %

[a]Dependent on underlying pathology, location of disease, and/or surgical preference

the time of pneumonectomy. **Chylothorax** can result from damage to the thoracic duct within the chest and occurs more commonly where there has been extensive mediastinal dissection, for example, during a mediastinal lymph node clearance for bronchogenic carcinoma or esophageal resection.

Major Complications

One of the most significant complications following pneumonectomy is **post-pneumonectomy pulmonary edema** in the remaining lung. This occurs more commonly following a right pneumonectomy and results from the significantly increased postoperatively pulmonary vascular resistance and subsequent cardiac compromise. This has a high mortality and is exceptionally difficult to treat. Fluid restriction post-pneumonectomy is successful in reducing the incidence of this complication. Another significant complication, particularly following left pneumonectomy, is that of **left recurrent laryngeal nerve injury**. This occurs as a result of the location of the left main pulmonary artery in relation to the aortic arch and recurrent laryngeal nerve, with dissection in this region resulting in direct nerve trauma. **Atrial fibrillation** occurs in over 20 % of patients following pneumonectomy. The incidence of atrial (and ventricular) arrhythmias has been significantly reduced by the use of thoracic epidural analgesia. **Pneumonia** following pneumonectomy is a serious complication and can result in **respiratory failure** and death. The incidence of this complication, too, has been reduced by thoracic epidural analgesia. **Empyema** and **abscess formation** are serious complications. Many patients will require a surgical drainage procedure, with the consequential debility this entails including prolonged hospital stay and other sequelae. Inadvertent **injury to the lung** is also possible especially in the presence of dense pleural adhesions, and occasionally, **pneumothorax** or **persistent air leak** may result. Complications specific to the underlying problem and reason for the lung resection, may occur. **Basal atelectasis** and sometimes secondary **lung infection** may also occur. **Chylothorax** and **bronchopleural fistula** formation are chronic debilitating problems that delay recovery significantly. **Multisystem organ failure** is extremely serious, the incidence being most related to the underlying lung pathology and other comorbidities, and is associated with **mortality** when it occurs.

Consent and Risk Reduction

Main Points to Explain

- Discomfort
- Bruising and bleeding
- Infection
- Pneumothorax (rare)
- Cardiac arrhythmias (usually minor)
- Failure of insertion
- Catheter displacement/later failure
- Further surgery

Further Reading, References, and Resources

Bronchoscopy

Baue AE. Glen's thoracic and cardiovascular surgery. 6th ed. Connecticut: Appleton and Lange; 1996

Sabiston DC, Spencer FC. Surgery of the chest. 5th ed. Philadelphia: WB Saunders; 1990.

Shields TW. General thoracic surgery. 4th ed. Baltimore: Williams & Wilkins; 1994.

Thoracoscopy

Baue AE. Glen's thoracic and cardiovascular surgery. 6th ed. Connecticut: Appleton and Lange; 1996

Clemente CD. Anatomy – a regional atlas of the human body. 4th ed. Baltimore: Williams and Wilkins; 1997.

Flores RM, Park BJ, Dycoco J, Aronova A, Hirth Y, Rizk NP, Bains M, Downey RJ, Rusch VW. Lobectomy by video-assisted thoracic surgery (VATS) versus thoracotomy for lung cancer. J Thorac Cardiovasc Surg. 2009;138(1):11–8.

Jamieson GG. The anatomy of general surgical operations. 2nd ed. Edinburgh: Churchill Livingston; 2006.

Nakanishi R, Oka S, Odate S. Video-assisted thoracic surgery major pulmonary resection requiring control of the main pulmonary artery. Interact Cardiovasc Thorac Surg. 2009;9(4):618–22. Epub 2009 Jul 14.

Sabiston DC, Spencer FC. Surgery of the chest. 5th ed. Philadelphia: WB Saunders; 1990.

Schuchert MJ, Pettiford BL, Pennathur A, Abbas G, Awais O, Close J, Kilic A, Jack R, Landreneau JR, Landreneau JP, Wilson DO, Luketich JD, Landreneau RJ. Anatomic segmentectomy for stage I non-small-cell lung cancer: comparison of video-assisted thoracic surgery versus open approach. J Thorac Cardiovasc Surg. 2009;138(6):1318–25.e1.

Seder CW, Hanna K, Lucia V, Boura J, Kim SW, Welsh RJ, Chmielewski GW. The safe transition from open to thoracoscopic lobectomy: a 5-year experience. Ann Thorac Surg. 2009;88(1): 216–25;discussion 225–6.

Shapiro M, Weiser TS, Wisnivesky JP, Chin C, Arustamyan M, Swanson SJ. Thoracoscopic segmentectomy compares favorably with thoracoscopic lobectomy for patients with small stage I lung cancer. J Thorac Cardiovasc Surg. 2009;137(6):1388–93. Epub 2009 Apr 11.

Shields TW. General thoracic surgery. 4th ed. Baltimore: Williams & Wilkins; 1994.

Yang X, Qu J, Wang S. Long-term outcomes of video-assisted thoracic surgery lobectomy for nonsmall cell lung cancer. South Med J. 2009;102(9):905–8.

Thoracotomy

Alifano M, Cusumano G, Strano S, Magdeleinat P, Bobbio A, Giraud F, Lebeau B, Régnard JF. Lobectomy with pulmonary artery resection: morbidity, mortality, and long-term survival. J Thorac Cardiovasc Surg. 2009;135(6):1400–5. Epub 2009 Feb 23.

Baue AE. Glen's thoracic and cardiovascular surgery. 6th ed. Connecticut: Appleton and Lange; 1996

Berry MF, Hanna J, Tong BC, Burfeind WR Jr, Harpole DH, D'Amico TA, Onaitis MW. Risk factors for morbidity after lobectomy for lung cancer in elderly patients. Ann Thorac Surg. 2009;88(4):1093–9.

Clemente CD. Anatomy – a regional atlas of the human body. 4th ed. Baltimore: Williams and Wilkins; 1997.

Jamieson GG. The anatomy of general surgical operations. 2nd ed. Edinburgh: Churchill Livingston; 2006.

Jichen QV, Chen G, Jiang G, Ding J, Gao W, Chen C. Risk factor comparison and clinical analysis of early and late bronchopleural fistula after non-small cell lung cancer surgery. Ann Thorac Surg. 2009;88(5):1589–93.

Kilic A, Schuchert MJ, Pettiford BL, Pennathur A, Landreneau JR, Landreneau JP, Luketich JD, Landreneau RJ. Anatomic segmentectomy for stage I non-small cell lung cancer in the elderly. Ann Thorac Surg. 2009;87(6):1662–6;discussion 1667–8.

Mansour Z, Kochetkova EA, Santelmo N, Meyer P, Wihlm JM, Quoix E, Massard G. Risk factors for early mortality and morbidity after pneumonectomy: a reappraisal. Ann Thorac Surg. 2009;88(6):1737–43.

Sabiston DC, Spencer FC. Surgery of the chest. 5th ed. Philadelphia: WB Saunders; 1990.

Seder CW, Hanna K, Lucia V, Boura J, Kim SW, Welsh RJ, Chmielewski GW. The safe transition from open to thoracoscopic lobectomy: a 5-year experience. Ann Thorac Surg. 2009;88(1):216–25;discussion 225–6.

Shields TW. General thoracic surgery. 4th ed. Baltimore: Williams & Wilkins; 1994.

Shrager JB, DeCamp MM, Murthy SC. Intraoperative and postoperative management of air leaks in patients with emphysema. Thorac Surg Clin. 2009;19(2):223–31, ix. Review.

Voltolini L, Rapicetta C, Ligabue T, Luzzi L, Scala V, Gotti G. Short- and long-term results of lung resection for cancer in octogenarians. Asian Cardiovasc Thorac Ann. 2009;17(2):147–52.

Partial Lung Resection

Alifano M, Cusumano G, Strano S, Magdeleinat P, Bobbio A, Giraud F, Lebeau B, Régnard JF. Lobectomy with pulmonary artery resection: morbidity, mortality, and long-term survival. J Thorac Cardiovasc Surg. 2009;137(6):1400–5.

Baue AE. Glen's thoracic and cardiovascular surgery. 6th ed. Connecticut: Appleton and Lange; 1996

Berry MF, Hanna J, Tong BC, Burfeind WR Jr, Harpole DH, D'Amico TA, Onaitis MW. Risk factors for morbidity after lobectomy for lung cancer in elderly patients. Ann Thorac Surg. 2009;88(4):1093–9.

Clemente CD. Anatomy – a regional atlas of the human body. 4th ed. Baltimore: Williams and Wilkins; 1997.

Ferguson MK, Gaissert HA, Grab JD, Sheng S. Pulmonary complications after lung resection in the absence of chronic obstructive pulmonary disease: the predictive role of diffusing capacity. J Thorac Cardiovasc Surg. 2009;138(6):1297–302

Flores RM, Park BJ, Dycoco J, Aronova A, Hirth Y, Rizk NP, Bains M, Downey RJ, Rusch VW. Lobectomy by video-assisted thoracic surgery (VATS) versus thoracotomy for lung cancer. J Thorac Cardiovasc Surg. 2009;138(1):11–8.

Jamieson GG. The anatomy of general surgical operations. 2nd ed. Edinburgh: Churchill Livingston; 2006.

Jichen QV, Chen G, Jiang G, Ding J, Gao W, Chen C. Risk factor comparison and clinical analysis of early and late bronchopleural fistula after non-small cell lung cancer surgery. Ann Thorac Surg. 2009;88(5):1589–93.

Kilic A, Schuchert MJ, Pettiford BL, Pennathur A, Landreneau JR, Landreneau JP, Luketich JD, Landreneau RJ. Anatomic segmentectomy for stage I non-small cell lung cancer in the elderly. Ann Thorac Surg. 2009;87(6):1662–6;discussion 1667–8.

Nakanishi R, Oka S, Odate S. Video-assisted thoracic surgery major pulmonary resection requiring control of the main pulmonary artery. Interact Cardiovasc Thorac Surg. 2009;9(4):618–22

Pettiford BL, Schuchert MJ, Abbas G, Pennathur A, Gilbert S, Kilic A, Landreneau JR, Jack R, Landreneau JP, Wilson DO, Luketich JD, Landreneau RJ. Anterior minithoracotomy: a direct approach to the difficult hilum for upper lobectomy, pneumonectomy, and sleeve lobectomy. Ann Surg Oncol. 2009. [Epub ahead of print].

Refai M, Brunelli A, Rocco G, Ferguson MK, Fortiparri SN, Salati M, La Rocca A, Kawamukai K. Does induction treatment increase the risk of morbidity and mortality after pneumonectomy? A multicentre case-matched analysis. Eur J Cardiothorac Surg. 2010;37(3):535–9.

Sabiston DC, Spencer FC. Surgery of the chest. 5th ed. Philadelphia:WB Saunders;1990.

Schuchert MJ, Pettiford BL, Pennathur A, Abbas G, Awais O, Close J, Kilic A, Jack R, Landreneau JR, Landreneau JP, Wilson DO, Luketich JD, Landreneau RJ. Anatomic segmentectomy for stage I non-small-cell lung cancer: comparison of video-assisted thoracic surgery versus open approach. J Thorac Cardiovasc Surg. 2009;138(6):1318–25.e1.

Seder CW, Hanna K, Lucia V, Boura J, Kim SW, Welsh RJ, Chmielewski GW. The safe transition from open to thoracoscopic lobectomy: a 5-year experience. Ann Thorac Surg. 2009;88(1): 216–25;discussion 225–6.

Shapiro M, Weiser TS, Wisnivesky JP, Chin C, Arustamyan M, Swanson SJ. Thoracoscopic segmentectomy compares favorably with thoracoscopic lobectomy for patients with small stage I lung cancer. J Thorac Cardiovasc Surg. 2009;137(6):1388–93

Shrager JB, DeCamp MM, Murthy SC. Intraoperative and postoperative management of air leaks in patients with emphysema. Thorac Surg Clin. 2009;19(2):223–31, ix. Review.

Shields TW. General thoracic surgery. 4th ed. Baltimore: Williams & Wilkins; 1994.

Voltolini L, Rapicetta C, Ligabue T, Luzzi L, Scala V, Gotti G. Short- and long-term results of lung resection for cancer in octogenarians. Asian Cardiovasc Thorac Ann. 2009;17(2):147–52.

Yang X, Qu J, Wang S. Long-term outcomes of video-assisted thoracic surgery lobectomy for nonsmall cell lung cancer. South Med J. 2009;102(9):905–8.

Total Pneumonectomy

Baue AE. Glen's thoracic and cardiovascular surgery. 6th ed. Connecticut: Appleton and Lange; 1996

Berry MF, Hanna J, Tong BC, Burfeind WR Jr, Harpole DH, D'Amico TA, Onaitis MW. Risk factors for morbidity after lobectomy for lung cancer in elderly patients. Ann Thorac Surg. 2009;88(4):1093–9.

Clemente CD. Anatomy – a regional atlas of the human body. 4th ed. Baltimore: Williams and Wilkins; 1997.

Ferguson MK, Gaissert HA, Grab JD, Sheng S. Pulmonary complications after lung resection in the absence of chronic obstructive pulmonary disease: the predictive role of diffusing capacity. J Thorac Cardiovasc Surg. 2009;138(6):1297–302. Epub 2009 Sep 26.

Jamieson GG. The anatomy of general surgical operations. 2nd ed. Edinburgh: Churchill Livingston; 2006.

Jichen QV, Chen G, Jiang G, Ding J, Gao W, Chen C. Risk factor comparison and clinical analysis of early and late bronchopleural fistula after non-small cell lung cancer surgery. Ann Thorac Surg. 2009;88(5):1589–93.

Mansour Z, Kochetkova EA, Santelmo N, Meyer P, Wihlm JM, Quoix E, Massard G. Risk factors for early mortality and morbidity after pneumonectomy: a reappraisal. Ann Thorac Surg. 2009;88(6):1737–43.

Nakanishi R, Oka S, Odate S. Video-assisted thoracic surgery major pulmonary resection requiring control of the main pulmonary artery. Interact Cardiovasc Thorac Surg. 2009;9(4):618–22. Epub 2009 Jul 14.

Pettiford BL, Schuchert MJ, Abbas G, Pennathur A, Gilbert S, Kilic A, Landreneau JR, Jack R, Landreneau JP, Wilson DO, Luketich JD, Landreneau RJ. Anterior minithoracotomy: a direct approach to the difficult hilum for upper lobectomy, pneumonectomy, and sleeve lobectomy. Ann Surg Oncol. 2010;17(1):123–8.

Refai M, Brunelli A, Rocco G, Ferguson MK, Fortiparri SN, Salati M, La Rocca A, Kawamukai K. Does induction treatment increase the risk of morbidity and mortality after pneumonectomy? A multicentre case-matched analysis. Eur J Cardiothorac Surg. 2010;37(3):535–9.

Sabiston DC, Spencer FC. Surgery of the chest. 5th ed. Philadelphia: WB Saunders; 1990.

Sahai RK, Nwogu CE, Yendamuri S, Tan W, Wilding GE, Demmy TL. Is thoracoscopic pneumonectomy safe? Ann Thorac Surg. 2009;88(4):1086–92.

Shields TW. General thoracic surgery. 4th ed. Baltimore: Williams & Wilkins; 1994.

Shrager JB, DeCamp MM, Murthy SC. Intraoperative and postoperative management of air leaks in patients with emphysema. Thorac Surg Clin. 2009;19(2):223–31, ix. Review.

Voltolini L, Rapicetta C, Ligabue T, Luzzi L, Scala V, Gotti G. Short- and long-term results of lung resection for cancer in octogenarians. Asian Cardiovasc Thorac Ann. 2009;17(2):147–52.

Chapter 8
Cardiac Surgery

James Edwards, Jayme Bennetts, and Brendon J. Coventry

General Perspective and Overview

The relative risks and complications increase proportionately according to the site, size, type, and complexity of the problem being addressed within the heart or chest and in relation to the age of the patient and other comorbidities. This is principally related to the surgical accessibility, ability to bypass coronary stenoses or replace valves, risk of other injury and respiratory compromise, functional reserve, technical ease, and the ability to achieve correction of the problem.

The main serious complications are **bleeding, myocardial infarction, thromboembolism, and infection,** which can be minimized by the adequate exposure, mobilization, technical care, optimal cardiopulmonary bypass, and avoiding lung injury and hematoma formation. Infection is the main sequel of tissue injury, respiratory obstruction, and hematoma formation and may arise from preexisting infection or be newly acquired. This can lead to **pleural infection, lung consolidation, abscess formation,** and **systemic sepsis. Multisystem failure** and **death** remain serious potential complications from cardiac surgery and systemic infection.

Neural injuries are not infrequent potential problems associated with cardiac surgery, because intercostal nerves travel beneath each rib and may be involved in rib mobilization, compression from retractors, scar formation, or even direct incision.

J. Edwards, MBBS, FRACS (✉)
Department of Surgery, Royal Adelaide Hospital, Adelaide, Australia
e-mail: jedwards@internode.on.net

J. Bennetts, BMBS, FRACS, FCSANZ
Cardiac and Thoracic Surgery, Flinders Medical Centre, Adelaide, Australia

B.J. Coventry, BMBS, PhD, FRACS, FACS, FRSM
Discipline of Surgery, Royal Adelaide Hospital, University of Adelaide,
L5 Eleanor Harrald Building, North Terrace, 5000 Adelaide, SA, Australia
e-mail: brendon.coventry@adelaide.edu.au

B.J. Coventry (ed.), *Cardio-Thoracic, Vascular, Renal and Transplant Surgery*,   125
Surgery: Complications, Risks and Consequences,
DOI 10.1007/978-1-4471-5418-1_8, © Springer-Verlag London 2014

Positioning on the operating table has been associated with increased risk of **deep venous thrombosis** and **nerve palsies**, especially in prolonged procedures. **Limb ischemia, compartment syndrome, and ulnar** and **common peroneal nerve palsy** are recognized potential complications, which should be checked for, as the patient's position may change during surgery.

Mortality associated with most cardiac surgery procedures is usually low and principally associated with pulmonary infarction or thromboembolism. Procedures involving the cardiac valves or coronary vessels during a major acute event (e.g., valve failure or myocardial infarction), or during acute respiratory compromise or concomitant with a cerebrovascular event, for example, carry higher risks associated with possible serious bleeding, infection, and other complications, including increased risk of mortality.

This chapter therefore attempts to draw together in one place the estimated overall frequencies of the complications associated with cardiac procedures, based on information obtained from the literature and experience. Not all patients are at risk of the full range of listed complications. It must be individualized for each patient and their disease process, but represents a guide and summary of the attendant risks, complications, and consequences.

With these factors and facts in mind, the information given in this chapter must be appropriately and discernibly interpreted and used.

Important Note

It should be emphasized that the risks and frequencies that are given here *represent derived figures*. These *figures are best estimates of relative frequencies across most institutions*, not merely the highest-performing ones, and as such are often representative of a number of studies, which include different patients with differing comorbidities and different surgeons. In addition, the risks of complications in lower or higher-risk patients may lie outside these estimated ranges, and individual clinical judgement is required as to the expected risks communicated to the patient, staff, or for other purposes. The range of risks is also derived from experience and the literature; while risks outside this range may exist, certain risks may be reduced or absent due to variations of procedures or surgical approaches. It is recognized that different patients, practitioners, institutions, regions, and countries may vary in their requirements and recommendations.

For complications related to other associated/additional surgery that may arise during cardiac surgery, see Chap. 7 Thoracic Surgery or the relevant volume and chapter.

The authors would like to thank Dr E Carmack Holmes, Sr, past Surgeon-in-Chief and Head of Cardiothoracic Surgery, UCLA, Los Angeles, USA, for discussion and advice.

Coronary Artery Bypass Grafting Surgery

Description

General anesthesia is used. The aim is to bypass an obstruction or stenosis in one or more coronary arteries using a segment of autologous vessel. A variety of vessel conduits may be selected for the donor graft, commonly including internal mammary artery, long saphenous vein, or radial artery and less commonly the short saphenous vein, gastroepiploic artery, or cephalic vein. The procedure is better used for proximal stenosis than very distal obstructions or diffuse disease. The approach is typically via a median sternotomy. Extracorporeal cardiac bypass circuits are most commonly used, although "off-pump" techniques are preferred in some centers. The sternum is usually closed using heavy wires and the skin sutured using subcuticular sutures.

Anatomical Points

The right and left main coronary arteries originate from the aortic root immediately after the aortic valve. The naming often varies slightly between texts; however, the terms "descending" and "interventricular" for the branches are synonymous. The *left coronary artery* arises from the left coronary sinus of Valsalva and divides to give off an anterior descending (interventricular) branch and then travels along the left atrioventricular groove as the circumflex artery, which supplies the posterior left ventricular wall. The right coronary artery passes along the right atrioventricular groove and branches into the marginal artery and posterior (inferior) descending (interventricular) artery, passing to the cardiac apex. Dominance of the coronary circulation refers to whether the left or right main coronary artery supplies the posterior descending (interventricular) coronary artery. In ~10 % of cases, the posterior as well as the anterior interventricular artery is a branch of the left coronary (a so-called "left dominant" system). The extent and sites of pathological stenosis can dictate the surgery required and the range and risk of complications. Other anatomic variations are possible.

Perspective

See Table 8.1. Coronary artery bypass graft (CABG) surgery in the modern era is routine, although it remains a major invasive procedure. However, the spectrum of cases presenting for coronary surgery becomes evermore complex, older, and with more comorbidities, influencing risk. Coronary arterial disease is a vascular disease, which is a generalized process, and patients presenting for CABG surgery are a high-risk group for multiple other complications. The risk of major

Table 8.1 Coronary artery bypass grafting surgery estimated frequency of complications, risks, and consequences

Complications, risks, and consequences	Estimated frequency
Most significant/serious complications	
Infection	
Subcutaneous/wound	1–5 %
Intrathoracic (pneumonia; pleural; empyema; abscess)	1–5 %
Mediastinitis	0.1–1 %
Osteomyelitis of sternum	1–5 %
Systemic	1–5 %
Bleeding and hematoma formation (intrathoracic; wound; hemothorax)	1–5 %
Reoperation for bleeding (acute <7 days)	1–5 %
Acute graft occlusion	1–5 %
Arrythmias (including AF)	20–50 %
Perioperative myocardial infarction	1–5 %
Cardiac failure	1–5 %
Respiratory failure and prolonged assisted ventilation[a]	1–5 %
Stroke (cerebrovascular accident)[a]	1–5 %
Altered psychological state/sleep disturbance/neurocognitive impairment	20–50 %
Graft failure rate (all causes at 10 years)	
Internal mammary artery graft	1–5 %
Other vessel grafts	20–50 %
Pulmonary embolism and deep venous thrombosis	1–5 %
Multisystem organ failure (renal, pulmonary, cardiac failure)[a]	1–5 %
Death[a]	1–5 %
Rare significant/serious problems	
Pericardial or pleural effusion (late)	0.1–1 %
Persistent air leak/pneumothorax (>48 h)	0.1–1 %
Gastrointestinal complications	0.1–1 %
Right thoracic duct injury (chylous leak, chylothorax, fistula)[a]	<0.1 %
Diaphragmatic injury/paresis	<0.1 %
Recurrent laryngeal nerve injury	<0.1 %
Esophageal injury[a]	<0.1 %
Less serious complications	
Saphenous vein donor site problems[a]	1–5 %
Surgical emphysema	0.1–1 %
Sternal wire protrusion/erosion/pain (median sternotomy)	1–5 %
Rib pain, wound pain (acute <4 weeks)	>80 %
Rib pain, wound pain (chronic >12 weeks)	1–5 %
Wound scarring problems	5–20 %
Deformity of rib/chest or skin (poor cosmesis)	1–5 %
Pleural drain tube(s)[a]	>80 %

[a]Dependent on underlying pathology, location of disease, surgical method, and/or surgical preference

complications is largely determined by the severity of the cardiac ischemic insult and comorbidities existing prior to surgery. Early major complications include death, bleeding, cardiac arrythmias, and wound infections. Chest infection is relatively common and is reduced by early mobilization and physiotherapy. Later, debilitating complications include sternal osteomyelitis and chronic pain, which are relatively rare but may be serious. Other major complications include respiratory, renal, and multiorgan failure, which may cause severe disability and prolong hospital stay, and are a significant cause of mortality. Postoperative instability of anticoagulation is relatively common, and bleeding from any site may result, but is rarely severe. Bleeding into the brain or gut may occur and can be catastrophic. Stroke may be embolic or associated with postoperative coagulopathy and is an early cause of mortality or serious permanent disability. Perioperative myocardial infarction may occur, as the underlying problem is coronary arterial insufficiency. The risks of CABG surgery have to be balanced against the risks of not performing the surgery, which may be considerable. CABG surgery is essentially palliative, and redo-CABG surgery is occasionally necessary, due to deterioration of the graft or progressive native coronary arterial disease. Other complications include discomfort, chronic pain, pulmonary embolism, and restenosis. Emergency operations carry higher risk than elective surgery. Carotid endarterectomy may need to precede CABG for high-grade carotid stenosis, to reduce stroke risk. Erosion of sternal wires through skin or dehiscence is alarming for the patient, although a relatively rare problem. Keloid scar formation may be severe, irritating, and unsightly. Insertion of pleural drain tubes is almost uniform.

Major Complications

Stroke, myocardial infarction, pulmonary embolus, pneumonia, intrathoracic bleeding, and severe arrhythmias represent serious complications which are fortunately rare but can be fatal or debilitating. **Altered mental function, DVT, infection, chronic pain, anticoagulation instability, reoperation, and sternal osteomyelitis** are usually less life-threatening but often severely debilitating complications. **Reoperation** may be required acutely (<7 days) most often due to bleeding or recurrent ischemia or chronically (>2 months) due to pericardial effusion, both being serious complications associated with increased morbidity and mortality. **Multisystem organ failure** prolongs ICU care and is the usual prodrome to **death** associated with complications of CABG, often related to underlying comorbidity. **Acute renal failure** may require dialysis and is associated with up to 50 % mortality. **Respiratory failure** may require prolonged mechanical ventilation. **Wound infection, sternal osteomyelitis, mediastinitis, and lung infection** are uncommon but can be serious complications. **Gastrointestinal complications** are rare and, when they arise, are often devastating. They may be severe including ulceration, bleeding, bowel ischemia, biliary colic/stasis, pseudo-obstruction/ileus, and pancreatitis. **Mortality** risk is increased (with or without operation) by existing preoperative conditions, such as diabetes, renal failure, cardiac failure, aortic disease, lung disease, advanced age, and recent smoking history. Significant risk of severe complications may occur without any surgery. Increased use of percutaneous revascularization methods may select out an older more complex population for CABG surgery, which may effectively increase the risk of complications, including mortality.

Consent and Risk Reduction

Main Points to Explain

- GA risk
- Wound infection
- Bleeding
- Cardiac arrythmias
- Stroke
- Respiratory infection
- Chest wall pain
- Respiratory or renal failure
- Further surgery, including reoperation
- Death

Aortic Valve Repair or Replacement Surgery

Description

General anesthesia is used. The aim is to replace or repair the malfunctioning aortic valve using a biological tissue or mechanical device or other repair method to re-create unencumbered unidirectional outflow. One of the main aims of cardiac surgery is to avoid the use of anticoagulants and the attendant risks of long-term use of these. Indications for anticoagulation in cardiac surgery include a mechanical prosthesis in any position (aortic, mitral, or tricuspid) or atrial fibrillation. Risks of long-term anticoagulation include thrombosis and embolism from under-anticoagulation and spontaneous bleeding (from brain, gut, and others) from over-anticoagulation. Aortic valve repair is a less commonly used technique and is being developed in a few specialized centers. The approach is typically via a median sternotomy. Extracorporeal cardiac bypass circuits are used. The sternum is usually closed using heavy wires and the skin sutured using subcuticular sutures.

Anatomical Points

The cusps of the aortic valve are usually free but may be fused, either congenitally or acquired. Patients with bicuspid aortic valves also have both an increased incidence of stenosis at a younger age and increased risk of an ascending aortic aneurysm. Other anatomical variants are possible.

Perspective

See Table 8.2. The most common problems associated with cardiac valve surgery are bleeding, cardiac arrhythmias, and chest infection. Infection is relatively rare but may be extremely severe if prosthetic-related endocarditis or sternal osteomyelitis

Table 8.2 Aortic valve repair or replacement surgery estimated frequency of complications, risks, and consequences

Complications, risks, and consequences	Estimated frequency
Most significant/serious complications	
Infection[a]	
Subcutaneous/wound	1–5 %
Intrathoracic (pneumonia; pleural)	1–5 %
Pulmonary empyema or abscess	0.1–1 %
Mediastinitis	0.1–1 %
Osteomyelitis of sternum	1–5 %
Systemic	1–5 %
Endocarditis (prosthetic valve)	0.1–1 %
Bleeding and hematoma formation (overall)[a]	1–5 %
Wound	0.1–1 %
Hemothorax	0.1–1 %
Pulmonary contusion	0.1–1 %
Peri-valvular leakage	1–5 %
Pulmonary embolism	1–5 %
Difficulty controlling anticoagulation[a]	5–20 %
Arrythmias	20–50 %
Conduction system injury/pacemaker requirement	1–5 %
Valve failure total[a]	5–20 %
Early (including para-valvular leak)	1–5 %
Late (all causes)	5–20 %
Hemolysis	1–5 %
Valve thrombosis	1–5 %
Cardiac failure	1–5 %
Perioperative myocardial infarction	1–5 %
Stroke (cerebrovascular accident)[a]	1–5 %
Altered psychological state/neurocognitive impairment/sleep disturbance (>2 months)	20–50 %
Reoperation for bleeding (acute <7 days)	1–5 %
Reoperation for prosthetic failure, thrombosis, infection (late)	5–20 %
Respiratory failure[a] and prolonged assisted ventilation[a]	1–5 %

(continued)

Table 8.2 (continued)

Complications, risks, and consequences	Estimated frequency
Multisystem organ failure (renal, pulmonary, cardiac failure)[a]	1–5 %
Death[a]	1–5 %
Rare significant/serious problems	
Persistent air leak/pneumothorax	0.1–1 %
Gastrointestinal complications	0.1–1 %
Aortic dissection	0.1–1 %
Pericardial effusion/tamponade (late)	0.1–1 %
Recurrent laryngeal nerve injury	<0.1 %
Esophageal injury[a]	<0.1 %
Diaphragmatic injury/paresis	<0.1 %
Thoracic duct injury (chylous leak, chylothorax, fistula)[a]	<0.1 %
Less serious complications	
Rib pain, wound pain (acute <4 weeks)	>80 %
Rib pain, wound pain (acute >12 weeks)	1–5 %
Sternal wire protrusion/erosion/pain (median sternotomy)	1–5 %
Surgical emphysema	0.1–1 %
Wound scarring problems	5–20 %
Deformity of rib/chest or skin (poor cosmesis)	1–5 %
Pleural drain tube(s)[a]	>80 %

[a]Dependent on underlying pathology, location of disease, and/or surgical preference

occurs. Anticoagulation difficulties postoperatively are also relatively common, and bleeding may result which may rarely be severe. Bleeding into the brain or gut may occur and can be catastrophic. Perioperative myocardial infarction may occur. Stroke may be a severe and serious problem. Other complications include discomfort, chronic pain, pulmonary embolism, and para-valvular leaks. Keloid scar formation may be severe, irritating, and unsightly. Emergency operations carry higher risk than elective surgery. Carotid endarterectomy may need to precede valve surgery for high-grade carotid stenosis, to reduce stroke risk. Erosion of sternal wires through skin or dehiscence, although a rare problem, is often alarming for the patient.

Major Complications

Stroke, myocardial infarction, pulmonary embolus, pneumonia, valve failure, intrathoracic bleeding, and severe arrhythmias represent serious complications which are fortunately rare but can be fatal. Aortic valve surgery necessarily requires manipulation close to the conduction system, especially in redo surgery, and **pacemaker insertion** may be required if injury to the conduction system occurs. **Altered mental function, DVT, chronic pain, anticoagulation instability, reoperation, and sternal osteomyelitis** are usually less life-threatening but often severely debilitating complications. **Reoperation** may be required acutely (<7 days) most often due to bleeding or chronically (>2 months) due to prosthetic failure; both are serious complications associated with increased morbidity and mortality. **Hemolysis** can be a severe problem often associated with para-valvular leakage. **Multisystem organ failure** prolongs ICU care and is the usual prodrome to death associated with complications of valve surgery, often related to underlying morbidity. **Renal failure** may require dialysis, and **pulmonary complications** may require prolonged mechanical ventilation. **Wound infection, sternal osteomyelitis, mediastinitis, lung infection,** and rarely **endocarditis** are uncommon but can be serious complications. **Gastrointestinal complications** are rare but may be severe including ulceration, bleeding, bowel ischemia, biliary colic/stasis, pseudo-obstruction/ileus, and pancreatitis. **Mortality** risk is increased (with or without operation) by existing preoperative comorbidities, such as diabetes, renal failure, cardiac failure, aortic disease, lung disease, advanced age, and recent smoking history. Significant risk of severe complications may occur without any surgery.

Consent and Risk Reduction

Main Points to Explain

- GA risk
- Wound infection
- Bleeding
- Cardiac arrythmias
- Pacemaker insertion
- Stroke
- Respiratory infection
- Chest wall pain
- Respiratory or renal failure
- Further surgery, including reoperation
- Death

Mitral Valve Repair or Replacement Surgery

Description

General anesthesia is used. The aim is to repair or replace the malfunctioning mitral valve using a variety of repair techniques or a biological tissue or mechanical device, to re-create unidirectional inflow to the ventricle. The approach is typically via a median sternotomy, although minimally invasive techniques are rapidly gaining favor. Mitral stenosis is more commonly rheumatic in origin and the valves are usually replaced, whereas mitral regurgitation has a variety of causes and the valves can usually be repaired. Competence of the mitral valve depends on the mitral annulus, valve leaflets, chordae tendineae, papillary muscles, and the left ventricular wall, so repair of the mitral valve is complex but in the modern era yields predictable results. Valve repair confers better survival figures than prosthetic replacement. One of the main aims of cardiac surgery is to avoid the use of anticoagulants and the attendant risks of long-term use of these. Indications for anticoagulation in cardiac surgery include a mechanical prosthesis in any position (aortic, mitral, or tricuspid) or atrial fibrillation. Risks of long-term anticoagulation include thrombosis and embolism from under-anticoagulation and spontaneous bleeding (from brain, gut, and others) from over-anticoagulation. Extracorporeal cardiac bypass circuits are used to allow entry to the heart. The sternum is usually closed using heavy wires and the skin sutured using subcuticular sutures.

Anatomical Points

The cusps of the mitral valve are usually free but may be fused, either congenitally or acquired. The pathology of the valve will largely determine the surgical technique and functional results.

Perspective

See Table 8.3. The most common problems associated with cardiac valve surgery are bleeding, prosthetic failure (short and long term), cardiac arrhythmias, and chest infection. Infection is relatively rare but may be extremely severe if

Table 8.3 Mitral valve repair or replacement surgery estimated frequency of complications, risks, and consequences

Complications, risks, and consequences	Estimated frequency
Most significant/serious complications	
Infection	
Subcutaneous/wound	1–5 %
Intrathoracic (pneumonia; pleural)	1–5 %
Osteomyelitis of sternum	1–5 %
Mediastinitis	0.1–1 %
Systemic	1–5 %
Endocarditis (prosthetic valve including late)	1–5 %
Peri-valvular leakage (immediate)	1–5 %
Valve failure total[a]	20–50 %
Early (including persistent regurgitation after repair)	1–5 %
Late (including prosthetic failure)	20–50 %
Arrythmias	20–50 %

Table 8.3 (continued)

Complications, risks, and consequences	Estimated frequency
Conduction system injury/pacemaker requirement	1–5 %
Bleeding and hematoma formation	1–5 %
Difficulty controlling anticoagulation	5–20 %
Hemolysis	1–5 %
Valve thrombosis	1–5 %
Rupture of valve ring (including A-V dehiscence and myocardial rupture)	1–5 %
Myocardial injury, cardiac failure, MI (hypotension)	1–5 %
Stroke (cerebrovascular accident)[a]	1–5 %
Altered psychological state/neurocognitive impairment, etc. (>2 months)	20–50 %
Reoperation (acute <7 days)	1–5 %
Reoperation (all causes; late >2 years)	20–50 %
Pulmonary embolism	1–5 %
Pulmonary failure[a]	1–5 %
Prolonged assisted ventilation[a]	1–5 %
Gastrointestinal complications	1–5 %
Multisystem organ failure (renal, pulmonary, cardiac failure)[a]	1–5 %
Death[a]	1–5 %
Rare significant/serious problems	
Pulmonary abscess and empyema	0.1–1 %
Pericardial effusion/tamponade	0.1–1 %
Recurrent laryngeal nerve injury	0.1–1 %
Esophageal injury[a]	0.1–1 %
Persistent air leak/pneumothorax/pulmonary injury	0.1–1 %
Bronchopleural fistula	0.1–1 %
Diaphragmatic injury/paresis	<0.1 %
Thoracic duct injury (chylous leak, fistula)[a]	<0.1 %
Less serious complications	
Rib pain, wound pain (acute <4 weeks)	>80 %
Rib pain, wound pain (acute >12 weeks)	1–5 %
Sternal wire protrusion/erosion/pain (median sternotomy)	1–5 %
Surgical emphysema	0.1–1 %
Wound scarring problems	5–20 %
Deformity of rib/chest or skin (poor cosmesis)	1–5 %
Pleural drain tube(s)[a]	>80 %

[a]Dependent on underlying pathology, location of disease, and/or surgical preference

prosthetic-related endocarditis or sternal osteomyelitis occurs. Anticoagulation difficulties postoperatively are also relatively common, but bleeding may result and may rarely be severe. Bleeding into the brain or gut may occur and can be catastrophic. Perioperative myocardial infarction may occur, as the underlying problem is cardiac insufficiency. Stroke may be a severe and serious debilitating problem. Other complications include discomfort, chronic pain, recurrent pneumothorax, pyothorax, pulmonary embolism, and restenosis/valve failure. Keloid scar formation may be severe, irritating, and unsightly. Emergency operations carry higher risk than elective surgery. Carotid endarterectomy may need to precede valve surgery for high-grade carotid stenosis, to reduce stroke risk. Erosion of sternal wires through skin or dehiscence is alarming for the patient, although a rare problem.

Major Complications

Stroke, myocardial infarction, pulmonary embolus, pneumonia, lung abscess, valve rupture, intrathoracic bleeding, and severe arrhythmias represent serious complications which are fortunately rare but can be fatal. Mitral valve surgery necessarily requires manipulation close to the conduction system, and **pacemaker insertion** may be required if injury to the conduction system occurs. **Altered mental function, DVT, infection, chronic pain, anticoagulation instability, reoperation, and sternal osteomyelitis** are usually less life-threatening but often severely debilitating complications. **Reoperation** may be required acutely (<7 days) most often due to bleeding or recurrent/persistent valve failure/rupture or chronically (>2 months) due to mechanical failure or restenosis; both are serious complications associated with increased morbidity and mortality. **Hemolysis** can be a severe problem. **Multisystem organ failure** prolongs ICU care and is the usual prodrome to **death** associated with complications of valve surgery, often related to underlying morbidity. **Renal failure** may require dialysis, and **pulmonary complications** may require prolonged mechanical ventilation. **Gastrointestinal complications** may be severe including ulceration, bleeding, bowel ischemia, biliary colic/stasis, pseudo-obstruction/ileus, and pancreatitis. **Mortality** risk is increased (with or without operation) by existing preoperative conditions, such as diabetes, renal failure, cardiac failure, aortic disease, lung disease, advanced age, and recent smoking history. Significant risk of severe complications may occur without any surgery.

Consent and Risk Reduction

Main Points to Explain

- GA risk
- Wound infection
- Bleeding
- Cardiac arrythmias
- Pacemaker insertion
- Stroke
- Respiratory infection
- Chest wall pain
- Respiratory or renal failure
- Further surgery, including reoperation
- Death

Tricuspid Valve Repair or Replacement Surgery

Description

General anesthesia is used. The aim is to replace or repair the malfunctioning tricuspid valve using a biological tissue or mechanical device or other repair method to re-create unidirectional flow. The approach is typically via a median sternotomy, although minimally invasive techniques are gaining considerable favor. Extracorporeal cardiac bypass circuits are used to allow entry to the heart. The sternum is usually closed using heavy wires and the skin sutured using subcuticular sutures.

Anatomical Points

The cusps of the tricuspid valve are considerably less well formed and more fragile and complex than the mitral. Competence of the tricuspid valve depends on the tricuspid annulus, valve leaflets, chordae tendineae, papillary muscles, and in particular on the morphology of the right ventricle, so repair of the tricuspid valve is complex and yields variable results. Results of replacement are also difficult to predict, often depending on postsurgical right ventricular performance. The anatomical orientation and pathology of the valve will largely determine the surgical technique and functional result.

Perspective

See Table 8.4. The most common problems associated with cardiac valve surgery are bleeding, mechanical failure (short and long term), cardiac arrhythmias, and chest infection. Infection is relatively rare but may be extremely severe if prosthetic-related endocarditis or sternal osteomyelitis occurs. Anticoagulation difficulties postoperatively are also relatively common, but bleeding may result and may rarely be severe. Bleeding into the brain or gut may occur and can be catastrophic. Perioperative myocardial infarction may occur, as the underlying problem is cardiac insufficiency. Stroke may be a severe and serious debilitating problem. Other complications include discomfort, chronic pain, recurrent pneumothorax, pyothorax, pulmonary embolism, and restenosis/valve failure. Keloid scar formation may be severe, irritating, and unsightly. Emergency operations carry higher risk than elective surgery. Carotid endarterectomy may need to precede valve surgery for high-grade carotid stenosis, to reduce stroke risk. Erosion of sternal wires through skin or dehiscence is alarming for the patient, although a rare problem.

Table 8.4 Tricuspid valve repair or replacement surgery estimated frequency of complications, risks, and consequences

Complications, risks, and consequences	Estimated frequency
Most significant/serious complications	
Infection	
Subcutaneous/wound	1–5 %
Intrathoracic (pneumonia; pleural)	1–5 %
Mediastinitis	0.1–1 %
Osteomyelitis of sternum	1–5 %
Systemic	1–5 %
Endocarditis (prosthetic valve)	1–5 %
Peri-valvular leakage	1–5 %
Valve failure total[a]	20–50 %
Early (including persistent regurgitation)	5–20 %
Late (including prosthetic failure)	5–20 %
Bleeding	1–5 %
Difficulty controlling anticoagulation	5–20 %
Arrythmias	20–50 %
Conduction system injury/pacemaker requirement	5–20 %
Myocardial injury, cardiac failure, MI (hypotension)	1–5 %
Stroke (cerebrovascular accident)[a]	1–5 %
Altered psychological state/neurocognitive impairment, etc. (>2 months)	20–50 %
Reoperation (acute <7 days)	1–5 %
Reoperation (late >2 years)	50–80 %
Pulmonary failure[a]	1–5 %
Prolonged assisted ventilation[a]	1–5 %
Gastrointestinal complications	1–5 %
Multisystem organ failure (renal, pulmonary, cardiac failure)[a]	1–5 %
Death[a]	1–5 %
Rare significant/serious problems	
Hematoma formation	
Wound	0.1–1 %
Hemothorax	0.1–1 %
Pulmonary contusion	0.1–1 %
Pericardial effusion/tamponade	0.1–1 %
Recurrent laryngeal nerve injury	0.1–1 %
Pulmonary embolism and venous thrombosis	0.1–1 %
Pulmonary empyema or abscess	0.1–1 %
Esophageal injury[a]	0.1–1 %
Persistent air leak/pneumothorax	0.1–1 %
Bronchopleural fistula	0.1–1 %
Pulmonary injury (direct or inferior pulmonary vein injury)	0.1–1 %
Diaphragmatic injury/paresis	<0.1 %
Thoracic duct injury (chylous leak, fistula)[a]	<0.1 %
Less serious complications	
Rib pain, wound pain (acute <4 weeks)	>80 %
Rib pain, wound pain (acute >12 weeks)	1–5 %
Sternal wire protrusion/erosion/pain (median sternotomy)	1–5 %
Surgical emphysema	0.1–1 %
Wound scarring problems	5–20 %

Table 8.4   (continued)

Complications, risks, and consequences	Estimated frequency
Deformity of rib/chest or skin (poor cosmesis)	1–5 %
Pleural drain tube(s)[a]	>80 %

[a]Dependent on underlying pathology, location of disease, and/or surgical preference

Major Complications

Stroke, myocardial infarction, pulmonary embolus, pneumonia, lung abscess, valve rupture, intrathoracic bleeding, and severe arrhythmias represent serious complications which are fortunately rare but can be fatal. Tricuspid valve surgery confers a particular risk to the conduction system, and **pacemaker insertion** is not uncommon if injury to the conduction system occurs. **Altered mental function, DVT, infection, chronic pain, anticoagulation instability, reoperation, and sternal osteomyelitis** are usually less life-threatening but often severely debilitating complications. **Reoperation** may be required acutely (<7 days) most often due to bleeding or recurrent/persistent valve failure/rupture or, chronically (>2 months), due to mechanical failure or restenosis; both are serious complications associated with increased morbidity and mortality. **Hemolysis** can be a severe problem. **Multisystem organ failure** prolongs ICU care and is the usual prodrome to **death** associated with complications of valve surgery, often related to underlying morbidity. **Renal failure** may require dialysis, and **pulmonary complications** may require prolonged mechanical ventilation. **Gastrointestinal complications** may be severe including ulceration, bleeding, bowel ischemia, biliary colic/stasis, pseudo-obstruction/ileus, and pancreatitis. **Mortality** risk is increased (with or without operation) by existing preoperative conditions, such as diabetes, renal failure, cardiac failure, aortic disease, lung disease, advanced age, and recent smoking history. Significant risk of severe complications may occur without any surgery.

Consent and Risk Reduction

Main Points to Explain

- GA risk
- Wound infection
- Bleeding
- Cardiac arrythmias
- Pacemaker insertion
- Stroke
- Respiratory infection
- Chest wall pain
- Respiratory or renal failure
- Death
- Further surgery, including reoperation

Further Reading, References, and Resources

Coronary Artery Bypass Grafting Surgery

Bagur R, Bertrand OF, Rodés-Cabau J, Rinfret S, Larose E, Tizón-Marcos H, Gleeton O, Nguyen CM, Roy L, Costerousse O, De Larochellière R. Comparison of outcomes in patients > or =70 years versus <70 years after transradial coronary stenting with maximal antiplatelet therapy for acute coronary syndrome. Am J Cardiol. 2009;104(5):624–9.

Baillot RG, Joanisse DR, Stevens LM, Doyle DP, Dionne B, Lellouche F. Recent evolution in demographic and clinical characteristics and in-hospital morbidity in patients undergoing coronary surgery. Can J Surg. 2009;52(5):394–400.

Baiou D, Karageorge A, Spyt T, Naylor AR. Patients undergoing cardiac surgery with asymptomatic unilateral carotid stenoses have a low risk of peri-operative stroke. Eur J Vasc Endovasc Surg. 2009;38(5):556–9.

Biancari F, Asim Mahar MA. Meta-analysis of randomized trials on the efficacy of posterior pericardiotomy in preventing atrial fibrillation after coronary artery bypass surgery. J Thorac Cardiovasc Surg. 2010;139(5):1158–61.

Brackbill ML, Sytsma CS, Sykes K. Perioperative outcomes of coronary artery bypass grafting: effects of metabolic syndrome and patient's sex. Am J Crit Care. 2009;18(5):468–73.

Bravata DM, Gienger AL, McDonald KM, Sundaram V, Perez MV, Varghese R, Kapoor JR, Ardehali R, Owens DK, Hlatky MA. Systematic review: the comparative effectiveness of percutaneous coronary interventions and coronary artery bypass graft surgery. Ann Intern Med. 2007;147(10):703–16.

Caplan LR. Translating what is known about neurological complications of coronary artery bypass graft surgery into action. Arch Neurol. 2009;66(9):1062–4.

Carey JS, Danielsen B, Milliken J, Li Z, Stabile BE. Narrowing the gap: early and intermediate outcomes after percutaneous coronary intervention and coronary artery bypass graft procedures in California, 1997 to 2006. J Thorac Cardiovasc Surg. 2009;138(5):1100–7.

Cartier R. Off-pump coronary artery revascularization in octogenarians: is it better? Curr Opin Cardiol. 2009;24(6):544–52.

Clemente CD. Anatomy – a regional atlas of the human body. 4th ed. Baltimore: Williams and Wilkins; 1997.

Curtis JP, Schreiner G, Wang Y, Chen J, Spertus JA, Rumsfeld JS, Brindis RG, Krumholz HM. All-cause readmission and repeat revascularization after percutaneous coronary intervention in a cohort of medicare patients. J Am Coll Cardiol. 2009;54(10):903–7.

De Hert S, Vlasselaers D, Barbé R, Ory JP, Dekegel D, Donnadonni R, Demeere JL, Mulier J, Wouters P. A comparison of volatile and non volatile agents for cardioprotection during on-pump coronary surgery. Anaesthesia. 2009;64(9):953–60.

Ghaferi AA, Birkmeyer JD, Dimick JB. Complications, failure to rescue, and mortality with major inpatient surgery in medicare patients. Ann Surg. 2009;250(6):1029–34.

Halkos ME, Puskas JD. Off-pump versus on-pump coronary artery bypass grafting. Surg Clin North Am. 2009;89(4):913–22. ix. Review.

Iribarne A, Karpenko A, Russo MJ, Cheema F, Umann T, Oz MC, Smith CR, Argenziano M. Eight-year experience with minimally invasive cardiothoracic surgery. World J Surg. 2010;34(4):611–5.

Ito N, Tashiro T, Morishige N, Iwahashi H, Nishimi M, Hayashida Y, Takeuchi K, Minematsu N, Kuwahara G, Sukehiro Y. Endoscopic radial artery harvesting for coronary artery bypass grafting: the initial clinical experience and results of the first 50 patients. Heart Surg Forum. 2009;12(6):E310–5.

Jamieson GG. The anatomy of general surgical operations. 2nd ed. Edinburgh: Churchill Livingston; 2006.

Jax TW, Peters AJ, Khattab AA, Heintzen MP, Schoebel FC. Percutaneous coronary revascularization in patients with formerly "refractory angina pectoris in end-stage coronary artery disease" – not "end-stage" after all. BMC Cardiovasc Disord. 2009;9:42.

Khan UA, Krishnamoorthy B, Najam O, Waterworth P, Fildes JE, Yonan N. A comparative analysis of saphenous vein conduit harvesting techniques for coronary artery bypass grafting–standard bridging versus the open technique. Interact Cardiovasc Thorac Surg. 2010;10(1):27–31.

Kim IC, Hur SH, Park NH, Jun DH, Cho YK, Nam CW, Kim H, Han SW, Choi SY, Kim YN, Kim KB. Incidence and predictors of silent embolic cerebral infarction following diagnostic coronary angiography. Int J Cardiol. 2011;148(2):179–82.

Kofidis T, Emmert MY, Paeschke HG, Emmert LS, Zhang R, Haverich A. Long-term follow-up after minimal invasive direct coronary artery bypass grafting procedure: a multi-factorial retrospective analysis at 1000 patient-years. Interact Cardiovasc Thorac Surg. 2009;9(6):990–4.

Kozower BD, Ailawadi G, Jones DR, Pates RD, Lau CL, Kron IL, Stukenborg GJ. Predicted risk of mortality models: surgeons need to understand limitations of the University HealthSystem Consortium models. J Am Coll Surg. 2009;209(5):551–6.

Li Y, Walicki D, Mathiesen C, Jenny D, Li Q, Isayev Y, Reed 3rd JF, Castaldo JE. Strokes after cardiac surgery and relationship to carotid stenosis. Arch Neurol. 2009;66(9):1091–6.

Litmathe J, Kurt M, Feindt P, Gams E, Boeken U. Predictors and outcome of ICU readmission after cardiac surgery. Thorac Cardiovasc Surg. 2009;57(7):391–4.

Liu YH, Wang DX, Li LH, Wu XM, Shan GJ, Su Y, Li J, Yu QJ, Shi CX, Huang YN, Sun W. The effects of cardiopulmonary bypass on the number of cerebral microemboli and the incidence of cognitive dysfunction after coronary artery bypass graft surgery. Anesth Analg. 2009;109(4):1013–22.

Mitrovic PM, Stefanovic B, Vasiljevic Z, Radovanovic M, Radovanovic N, Krljanac G, Novakovic A, Ostojic M. In-hospital and long-term prognosis after myocardial infarction in patients with prior coronary artery bypass surgery; 19-year experience. Sci World J. 2009;9:1023–30.

Moller JH, Shumway SJ, Gott VL. The first open-heart repairs using extracorporeal circulation by cross-circulation: a 53-year follow-up. Ann Thorac Surg. 2009;88(3):1044–6.

Paul S, Altorki NK, Port JL, Stiles BM, Lee PC. Surgical management of chylothorax. Thorac Cardiovasc Surg. 2009;57(4):226–8.

Prapas SN, Panagiotopoulos IA, Pentchev DN, Ayyad MA, Protogeros DA, Kotsis VN, Linardakis IN, Tzanavaras TP, Stratigi PT. Aorta no-touch off-pump coronary artery revascularization in octogenarians: 5 years' experience. Heart Surg Forum. 2009;12(6):E349–53.

Shen Y, Drum M, Roth S. The prevalence of perioperative visual loss in the United States: a 10-year study from 1996 to 2005 of spinal, orthopedic, cardiac, and general surgery. Anesth Analg. 2009;109(5):1534–45.

Silva J, Maroto LC, Rodríguez E. Multiple procedures for coronary disease: a surgeon's perspective from the operating theatre. Euro Intervent. 2009;5(Suppl D):D34–6.

Siminelakis S, Kotsanti A, Siafakas M, Dimakopoulos G, Sismanidis S, Koutentakis M, Paziouros C, Papadopoulos G. Is there any difference in carotid stenosis between male and female patients undergoing coronary artery bypass grafting? Interact Cardiovasc Thorac Surg. 2009;9(5):823–6.

Toor I, Bakhai A, Keogh B, Curtis M, Yap J. Age > or =75 years is associated with greater resource utilization following coronary artery bypass grafting. Interact Cardiovasc Thorac Surg. 2009;9(5):827–31.

Aortic Valve Repair or Replacement Surgery

Aicher D, Fries R, Rodionycheva S, Schmidt K, Langer F, Schäfers HJ. Aortic valve repair leads to a low incidence of valve-related complications. Eur J Cardiothorac Surg. 2010;37(1):127–32.

Brecht R, Friedrich M, Heinisch PP, Plonien K, Akra B, Hagl C, Khoynezhad A, Lutter G, Bombien R. Transcatheter valve replacement: new concepts for microsurgery inside the heart. Innovations (Phila). 2013;8(1):29–36.

Chikwe J, Croft LB, Goldstone AB, Castillo JG, Rahmanian PB, Adams DH, Filsoufi F. Comparison of the results of aortic valve replacement with or without concomitant coronary artery bypass grafting in patients with left ventricular ejection fraction <or=30% versus patients with ejection fraction >30%. Am J Cardiol. 2009;104(12):1717–21.

Clemente CD. Anatomy – a regional atlas of the human body. 4th ed. Baltimore: Williams and Wilkins; 1997.

Ghaferi AA, Birkmeyer JD, Dimick JB. Complications, failure to rescue, and mortality with major inpatient surgery in medicare patients. Ann Surg. 2009;250(6):1029–34.

Halkos ME, Chen EP, Sarin EL, Kilgo P, Thourani VH, Lattouf OM, Vega JD, Morris CD, Vassiliades T, Cooper WA, Guyton RA, Puskas JD. Aortic valve replacement for aortic stenosis in patients with left ventricular dysfunction. Ann Thorac Surg. 2009;88(3):746–51.

Iribarne A, Karpenko A, Russo MJ, Cheema F, Umann T, Oz MC, Smith CR, Argenziano M. Eight-year experience with minimally invasive cardiothoracic surgery. World J Surg. 2010;34(4):611–5.

Jamieson GG. The anatomy of general surgical operations. 2nd ed. Edinburgh: Churchill Livingston; 2006.

Lapar DJ, Yang Z, Stukenborg GJ, Peeler BB, Kern JA, Kron IL, Ailawadi G. Outcomes of reoperative aortic valve replacement after previous sternotomy. J Thorac Cardiovasc Surg. 2010;139(2):263–72.

Plass A, Scheffel H, Alkadhi H, Kaufmann P, Genoni M, Falk V, Grünenfelder J. Aortic valve replacement through a minimally invasive approach: preoperative planning, surgical technique, and outcome. Ann Thorac Surg. 2009;88(6):1851–6.

Mitral Valve Repair or Replacement Surgery

Caimmi PP, Diterlizzi M, Grossini E, Kapetanakis EI, Gavinelli M, Carriero A, Vacca G. Impact of prosthetic mitral rings on aortomitral apparatus function: a cardiac magnetic resonance imaging study. Ann Thorac Surg. 2009;88(3):740–4.

Casselman FP, La Meir M, Jeanmart H, Mazzarro E, Coddens J, Van Praet F, Wellens F, Vermeulen Y, Vanermen H. Endoscopic mitral and tricuspid valve surgery after previous cardiac surgery. Circulation. 2007;116 Suppl 11:I270–5

Clemente CD. Anatomy – a regional atlas of the human body. 4th ed. Baltimore: Williams and Wilkins; 1997.

Ghaferi AA, Birkmeyer JD, Dimick JB. Complications, failure to rescue, and mortality with major inpatient surgery in medicare patients. Ann Surg. 2009;250(6):1029–34.

Hill KM. Surgical repair of cardiac valves. Crit Care Nurs Clin North Am. 2007;19(4):353–60. v. Review.

Iribarne A, Karpenko A, Russo MJ, Cheema F, Umann T, Oz MC, Smith CR, Argenziano M. Eight-year experience with minimally invasive cardiothoracic surgery. World J Surg. 2010;34(4):611–5

Jamieson GG. The anatomy of general surgical operations. 2nd ed. Edinburgh: Churchill Livingston; 2006.

Kim JB, Kim HJ, Moon DH, Jung SH, Choo SJ, Chung CH, Song H, Lee JW. Long-term outcomes after surgery for rheumatic mitral valve disease: valve repair versus mechanical valve replacement. Eur J Cardiothorac Surg. 2010;37(5):1039–46.

Luciani GB, Viscardi F, Pilati M, Barozzi L, Faggian G, Mazzucco A. Operative risk and outcome of surgery in adults with congenital valve disease. ASAIO J. 2008;54(5):458–62.

Stingl C, Moller JH, Binstadt BA. Cardiac operations for North American children with rheumatic diseases: 1985–2005. Pediatr Cardiol. 2010;31(1):66–73.

Verbrugghe P, Meuris B, Flameng W, Herijgers P. Reconstruction of atrioventricular valves with photo-oxidized bovine pericardium. Interact Cardiovasc Thorac Surg. 2009;9(5):775–9.

Tricuspid Valve Repair or Replacement Surgery

Bernal JM, Pontón A, Diaz B, Llorca J, García I, Sarralde A, Diago C, Revuelta JM. Surgery for rheumatic tricuspid valve disease: a 30-year experience. J Thorac Cardiovasc Surg. 2008;136(2):476–81. Epub 2008 Jun 12.

Casselman FP, La Meir M, Jeanmart H, Mazzarro E, Coddens J, Van Praet F, Wellens F, Vermeulen Y, Vanermen H. Endoscopic mitral and tricuspid valve surgery after previous cardiac surgery. Circulation. 2007;116 Suppl 11:I270–5.

Chan V, Burwash IG, Lam BK, Auyeung T, Tran A, Mesana TG, Ruel M. Clinical and echocardiographic impact of functional tricuspid regurgitation repair at the time of mitral valve replacement. Ann Thorac Surg. 2009;88(4):1209–15.

Clemente CD. Anatomy – a regional atlas of the human body. 4th ed. Baltimore: Williams and Wilkins; 1997.

Dandekar U, Sachithanandan A, Kalkat M, Ridley P, Satur CM. Isolated severe ischemic tricuspid regurgitation: successful surgical repair. J Heart Valve Dis. 2007;16(3):331–2.

Gatti G, Marcianò F, Antonini-Canterin F, Pinamonti B, Benussi B, Pappalardo A, Zingone B. Tricuspid valve annuloplasty with a flexible prosthetic band. Interact Cardiovasc Thorac Surg. 2007;6(6):731–5.

Guenther T, Noebauer C, Mazzitelli D, Busch R, Tassani-Prell P, Lange R. Tricuspid valve surgery: a thirty-year assessment of early and late outcome. Eur J Cardiothorac Surg. 2008;34(2):402–9. discussion 409.

Hill KM. Surgical repair of cardiac valves. Crit Care Nurs Clin North Am. 2007;19(4):353–60. v. Review..

Iscan ZH, Vural KM, Bahar I, Mavioglu L, Saritas A. What to expect after tricuspid valve replacement? Long-term results. Eur J Cardiothorac Surg. 2007;32(2):296–300.

Jamieson GG. The anatomy of general surgical operations. 2nd ed. Edinburgh: Churchill Livingston; 2006.

Luciani GB, Viscardi F, Pilati M, Barozzi L, Faggian G, Mazzucco A. Operative risk and outcome of surgery in adults with congenital valve disease. ASAIO J. 2008;54(5):458–62.

Moraca RJ, Moon MR, Lawton JS, Guthrie TJ, Aubuchon KA, Moazami N, Pasque MK, Damiano Jr RJ. Outcomes of tricuspid valve repair and replacement: a propensity analysis. Ann Thorac Surg. 2009;87(1):83–8. discussion 88–9.

Park CK, Park PW, Sung K, Lee YT, Kim WS, Jun TG. Early and midterm outcomes for tricuspid valve surgery after left-sided valve surgery. Ann Thorac Surg. 2009;88(4):1216–23.

Scherptong RW, Vliegen HW, Winter MM, Holman ER, Mulder BJ, van der Wall EE, Hazekamp MG. Tricuspid valve surgery in adults with a dysfunctional systemic right ventricle: repair or replace? Circulation. 2009;119(11):1467–72.

Tang H, Xu Z, Zou L, Han L, Lu F, Lang X, Song Z. Valve repair with autologous pericardium for organic lesions in rheumatic tricuspid valve disease. Ann Thorac Surg. 2009;87(3):726–30.

Verbrugghe P, Meuris B, Flameng W, Herijgers P. Reconstruction of atrioventricular valves with photo-oxidized bovine pericardium. Interact Cardiovasc Thorac Surg. 2009;9(5):775–9.

Yang X, Wu Q, Xu J, Shen X, Gao S, Liu F. Repair of flail leaflet of the tricuspid valve by a simple cusp remodeling technique. J Card Surg. 2007;22(4):333–5.

Additional Reading, References, and Resources

Al Jaaly E, Fiorentino F, Reeves BC, Ind PW, Angelini GD, Kemp S, Shiner RJ. Effect of adding postoperative noninvasive ventilation to usual care to prevent pulmonary complications in patients undergoing coronary artery bypass grafting: a randomized controlled trial. J Thorac Cardiovasc Surg. 2013;146(4):912–8.

Alexander JH. Clinical-outcome trials in cardiac surgery–have we primed the pump? N Engl J Med. 2013;368(13):1247–8.

Comparing the effectiveness of coronary artery bypass graft surgery and nonsurgical catheter-based interventions for coronary artery disease. Ann Intern Med. 2013. [Epub ahead of print] [No authors listed].

Diegeler A, Börgermann J, Kappert U, Breuer M, Böning A, Ursulescu A, Rastan A, Holzhey D, Treede H, Rieß FC, Veeckmann P, Asfoor A, Reents W, Zacher M, Hilker M. GOPCABE study group off-pump versus on-pump coronary-artery bypass grafting in elderly patients. N Engl J Med. 2013;368(13):1189–98.

Farkouh ME, Domanski M, Sleeper LA, Siami FS, Dangas G, Mack M, Yang M, Cohen DJ, Rosenberg Y, Solomon SD, Desai AS, Gersh BJ, Magnuson EA, Lansky A, Boineau R, Weinberger J, Ramanathan K, Sousa JE, Rankin J, Bhargava B, Buse J, Hueb W, Smith CR, Muratov V, Bansilal S, King 3rd S, Bertrand M, Fuster V. FREEDOM trial investigators strategies for multivessel revascularization in patients with diabetes. N Engl J Med. 2012;367(25):2375–84.

Farkouh ME, Domanski M, Fuster V. Revascularization strategies in patients with diabetes. N Engl J Med. 2013;368(15):1455–6.

Head SJ, Kappetein AP. Off-pump or on-pump coronary-artery bypass grafting. N Engl J Med. 2012;367(6):577–8. author reply 578.

Hlatky MA. Compelling evidence for coronary-bypass surgery in patients with diabetes. N Engl J Med. 2012;367(25):2437–8.

Hlatky MA, Boothroyd DB, Baker L, Kazi DS, Solomon MD, Chang TI, Shilane D, Go AS. Comparative effectiveness of multivessel coronary bypass surgery and multivessel percutaneous coronary intervention: a cohort study. Ann Intern Med. 2013;158(10):727–34.

Khadka J, McAlinden C, Pesudovs K. Cognitive trajectories after postoperative delirium. N Engl J Med. 2012;367(12):1164. author reply 1164–5.

Kirtane AJ, Pinto DS, Moses JW. Comparative effectiveness of revascularization strategies. N Engl J Med. 2012;367(5):476.

Lamy A, Devereaux PJ, Prabhakaran D, Taggart DP, Hu S, Paolasso E, Straka Z, Piegas LS, Akar AR, Jain AR, Noiseux N, Padmanabhan C, Bahamondes JC, Novick RJ, Vaijyanath P, Reddy SK, Tao L, Olavegogeascoechea PA, Airan B, Sulling TA, Whitlock RP, Ou Y, Pogue J, Chrolavicius S, Yusuf S. Coronary investigators effects of off-pump and on-pump coronary-artery bypass grafting at 1 year. N Engl J Med. 2013;368(13):1179–88.

Le Strat Y. Cognitive trajectories after postoperative delirium. N Engl J Med. 2012;367(12):1164. author reply 1164-5.

Navia D, Vrancic M, Piccinini F, Camporrotondo M, Thierer J, Gil C, Benzadon M. Is the second internal thoracic artery better than the radial artery in total arterial off-pump coronary artery bypass grafting? A propensity score-matched follow-up study. J Thorac Cardiovasc Surg. 2013. pii: S0022-5223(13)00162-1. [Epub ahead of print].

Polomsky M, He X, O'Brien SM, Puskas JD. Outcomes of off-pump versus on-pump coronary artery bypass grafting: impact of preoperative risk. J Thorac Cardiovasc Surg. 2013 May;145(5):1193–8.

Sobolev BG, Fradet G, Kuramoto L, Rogula B. The occurrence of adverse events in relation to time after registration for coronary artery bypass surgery: a population-based observational study. J Cardiothorac Surg. 2013;8(1):74.

Thiele H, Zeymer U, Neumann FJ, Ferenc M, Olbrich HG, Hausleiter J, Richardt G, Hennersdorf M, Empen K, Fuernau G, Desch S, Eitel I, Hambrecht R, Fuhrmann J, Böhm M, Ebelt H, Schneider S, Schuler G, Werdan K, IABP-SHOCK II Trial Investigators. Intraaortic balloon support for myocardial infarction with cardiogenic shock. N Engl J Med. 2012;367(14):1287–96.

Usta E, Elkrinawi R, Ursulescu A, Nagib R, Mädge M, Salehi-Gilani S, Franke UF. Clinical outcome and quality of life after reoperative CABG: off-pump versus on-pump – observational pilot study. J Cardiothorac Surg. 2013;8:66.

Weintraub WS, Grau-Sepulveda MV, Weiss JM, O'Brien SM, Peterson ED, Kolm P, Zhang Z, Klein LW, Shaw RE, McKay C, Ritzenthaler LL, Popma JJ, Messenger JC, Shahian DM, Grover FL, Mayer JE, Shewan CM, Garratt KN, Moussa ID, Dangas GD, Edwards FH. Comparative effectiveness of revascularization strategies. N Engl J Med. 2012;366(16):1467–76.

Wittwer T, Sabashnikov A, Rahmanian PB, Choi YH, Zeriouh M, Mehler TO, Wahlers T. Less invasive coronary artery revascularization with a minimized extracorporeal circulation system: preliminary results of a comparative study with off-pump-procedures. J Cardiothorac Surg. 2013;8(1):75.

Chapter 9
Renal Surgery

John Miller, Oliver Hakenberg, Villis Marshall, and Brendon J. Coventry

General Perspective and Overview

Renal surgery has developed rapidly over the last 20 years, principally with the advent of laparoscopic procedures, lithotripsy and even robotic surgery. Many residents "cut their teeth" on ureterolithotomy in the age of open surgery, much as they did with open appendicectomy. Complete nephrectomy was traditionally practiced by more experienced surgeons and remains the principal therapy for malignant conditions affecting the kidney and collecting system, but the practice of selective partial nephrectomy is allowing preservation of partial renal function in highly selected settings in institutions where the facilities exist and surgeons are familiar with these techniques.

Partial nephrectomy is almost internationally now the standard treatment for all renal tumors <4 cm in size, and perhaps up to 5 cm, according to European, American, and Australian guidelines, and laparoscopic nephrectomy is considered standard treatment for all other tumors except complicated ones (T4). Open nephrectomy for tumors >10 cm in size is the usual standard approach; otherwise laparoscopic nephrectomy is widely used. The robotic approach is now becoming more popular where available and appropriate.

J. Miller, MBBS FRACS(Urology) (✉)
Department of Surgery, Queen Elizabeth Hospital, Adelaide, Australia
e-mail: urology@internode.on.net

O. Hakenberg, MD, PhD
Department of Urology, University Hospital, Rostock University, Rostock, Germany

V. Marshall, MD, FRACS
Discipline of Surgery, The University of Adelaide,
Royal Adelaide Hospital, Adelaide, Australia

B.J. Coventry, BMBS, PhD, FRACS, FACS, FRSM
Discipline of Surgery, Royal Adelaide Hospital, University of Adelaide,
L5 Eleanor Harrald Building, North Terrace, 5000 Adelaide, SA, Australia
e-mail: brendon.coventry@adelaide.edu.au

B.J. Coventry (ed.), *Cardio-Thoracic, Vascular, Renal and Transplant Surgery*,
Surgery: Complications, Risks and Consequences,
DOI 10.1007/978-1-4471-5418-1_9, © Springer-Verlag London 2014

With these factors and facts in mind, the information given in these chapters must be appropriately and discernibly interpreted and used.

The **use of specialized units with standardized preoperative assessment, multidisciplinary input, and high-quality postoperative care** is essential to the success of complex renal surgery overall and can significantly reduce risk of complications or aid early detection and prompt intervention.

Important Note

It should be emphasized that the risks and frequencies that are given here *represent derived figures.* These *figures are best estimates of relative frequencies across most institutions*, not merely the highest-performing ones, and as such are often representative of a number of studies, which include different patients with differing comorbidities and different surgeons. In addition, the risks of complications in lower or higher-risk patients may lie outside these estimated ranges, and individual clinical judgement is required as to the expected risks communicated to the patient, staff, or for other purposes. The range of risks is also derived from experience and the literature; while risks outside this range may exist, certain risks may be reduced or absent due to variations of procedures or surgical approaches. It is recognized that different patients, practitioners, institutions, regions, and countries may vary in their requirements and recommendations.

Nephrectomy or Partial Nephrectomy

Description

General anesthesia is used. The usual indications for a nephrectomy are a renal cell or urothelial carcinoma. Benign indications are an end-stage kidney disease with renal hypertension, a nonfunctioning atrophic kidney, an obstructed kidney with recurrent infections, a multicystic kidney disease with symptoms, or a living-related transplant donor nephrectomy. Indications for partial nephrectomy are small renal tumors or nonfunctioning segments of duplex kidneys. Partial nephrectomy is almost internationally now the standard treatment for all renal tumors <4 cm in size, and perhaps up to 5 cm, according to European, American, and Australian guidelines, and laparoscopic nephrectomy is considered standard treatment for all other tumors except complicated ones (T4). Open nephrectomy for tumors >10 cm in size is the usual standard approach; otherwise laparoscopic nephrectomy is widely used. The robotic approach is now becoming more popular where available and appropriate.

The aim of the procedure is to remove the affected kidney (totally or partially). Complete removal of the ureter is only necessary in upper tract urothelial carcinoma or with distended ureters in duplex kidneys. Removal of a surrounding bladder cuff around the vesicoureteric junction may be required. Surgery is determined by the extent of disease, but resection of the kidney and the upper ureter is usual, with surrounding lymph nodes. If infiltration of other organs in large renal tumors is present (spleen, tail of pancreas, hemicolon), these need to be removed en bloc with the kidney. The extent of resection and consequent complications are largely determined by the extent of disease. The approach used depends on the pathology, lesion size, required access, and often surgeon preference and expertise. A retroperitoneal lumbar approach by a lateral flank incision in the line of the 11th or 12th rib is usually used. For large tumors, a transperitoneal approach by a chevron, midline, or pararectal (paramedian) incision (or occasionally a thoracoabdominal incision) gives better exposure. Large renal tumors with tumor thrombus extension into the vena cava require excellent exposure and mobilization of the liver. Partial nephrectomy has been used with excellent outcomes for benign and malignant renal tumors of less than 4 cm in diameter. Open partial nephrectomy without lymphadenectomy is now the standard treatment for T1a renal cell carcinomas. The incision is typically mass-closed and the skin is closed with absorbable subcuticular interrupted sutures.

Anatomical Points

The kidneys develop as three successive sets of organs between the 4th and 8th week of gestation and migrate to about the L1 level by birth. Both kidneys may be joined anteriorly, forming a single horseshoe kidney, or each kidney may be segmented with separate ureteric drainage and/or vascular supply. Duplex ureteric systems are not uncommon. Ectopic kidneys also occur as well as unilateral renal agenesis. Congenital anomalies of the renal system may result in vesicoureteric reflux and/or renal failure. The anatomical extent of a renal tumor and the displacement or involvement of adjacent organs largely determines the surgery required, and this may be reasonably planned preoperatively using ultrasound and CT or MRI.

Perspective

See Table 9.1. For tumors confined within Gerota's fascia, the procedure is relatively well defined and, overall, carries little risk. For more advanced tumors, extensive surgery is associated with a higher risk of complications. Severe bleeding and injury to adjacent structures can occur but are uncommon. Injury to the pancreas that is unrecognized during surgery may invoke pancreatitis or pancreatic leakage, leading to a pancreatic collection, which may become infected and sometimes form an external fistula. Seromas are not uncommon, but lymphatic collections are; both may not be symptomatic, unless they are large, compress other structures, or become infected. Small bowel obstruction due to postoperative adhesions is very uncommon but does occur after transperitoneal surgery.

Table 9.1 Nephrectomy or partial nephrectomy estimated frequency of complications, risks, and consequences

Complications, risks, and consequences	Estimated frequency
Most significant/serious complications	
Infection[a]	
Subcutaneous/wound	1–5 %
Urinary/systemic	1–5 %
Chest infection	1–5 %
Basal atelectasis	5–20 %
Bleeding/hematoma/seroma/lymphocele/lymph ascites/fistula[b]	1–5 %
Paralytic ileus[b]	
With flank approach	0.1–1 %
With transabdominal approach	1–5 %
Renal impairment	5–20 %
Urine leakage/collection (urinoma)[a]	1–5 %
Small bowel obstruction (early or late)[a]	0.1–1 %
Rare significant/serious problems	
Pancreatitis/pancreatic injury/cyst/leakage/fistula	0.1–1 %
Bowel injury (stomach, duodenum, small bowel, colon)[b]	<0.1 %
Diaphragmatic injury[a]	<0.1 %
Deep venous thrombosis/pulmonary embolism	0.1–1 %
Splenectomy[a,b,c]	0.1–1 %
Multisystem organ failure[a]	0.1–1 %
Death[a]	<0.1 %
Less serious complications	
Pain/discomfort/tenderness	
Short term (<4 weeks)	20–50 %
Longer term (>12 weeks)	0.1–1 %
Nerve injury/sensory changes (lumbar plexus/branches/sympathetic chain)[a]	1–5 %
Urinary retention/catheterization	0.1–1 %
Wound scarring (deformity/dimpling of wound scar/poor cosmesis)	1–5 %
Incisional hernia (avoid lifting/straining for 8 weeks)	1–5 %
Drain tube(s)[a]	5–20 %

[a]Dependent on underlying pathology, surgical technique preferences, incision used, and location on the body
[b]Incidence may be higher for large or extensive masses
[c]Splenic preservation may sometimes be possible for splenic traumatic injury

Major Complications/Consequences

Bleeding is one of the major potential complications of nephrectomy. **Transfusion** is rarely required for nephrectomy. Slow ooze and either **seroma** or **hematoma formation** can occur and may develop **secondary infection** and **abscess formation**. **Wound infection** and rarely **wound dehiscence** can result in later **incisional hernia formation**. Infection may occasionally lead to **systemic sepsis** and even **multisystem organ failure**, which is a significant cause of early **mortality** when it occurs. Later mortality is due to **tumor recurrence or persistence**. Splenic injury and **splenectomy** are rare complications with left nephrectomy, largely dependent on tumor extension. Significant **lymphatic leakage** may very rarely occur from **thoracic duct injury**, which will lead to **lymphatic ascites or collection**. **Small bowel obstruction** may be a recurrent issue after transperitoneal nephrectomy, often treated well conservatively, but surgery may be required.

Consent and Risk Reduction

Main Points to Explain

- GA risk
- Bleeding/hematoma
- Infection (local/systemic)
- Respiratory complications
- Deep venous thrombosis/pulmonary embolism
- Pain/discomfort
- Possible tumor recurrence*
- Urine leakage*
- Urine collection*
- Other abdominal organ injury
- Possible blood transfusion
- Renal impairment
- Risks without surgery

*Dependent on pathology and type of surgery performed

Laparoscopic Nephrectomy or Laparoscopic Partial Nephrectomy

Description

General anesthesia is used. The usual indications for a laparoscopic nephrectomy or laparoscopic partial nephrectomy are renal cell carcinoma and, rarely, a benign end-stage kidney disease with a nonfunctioning kidney. Partial nephrectomy is almost internationally now the standard treatment for all renal tumors <4 cm in size, and perhaps up to 5 cm, according to European, American, and Australian guidelines, and laparoscopic nephrectomy is considered standard treatment for all other tumors except complicated ones (T4). Open nephrectomy for tumors >10 cm in size is the usual standard approach; otherwise laparoscopic nephrectomy is widely used. The robotic approach is now becoming more popular where available and appropriate.

   The aim of the procedure is to remove the affected kidney or the tumor-bearing part of the kidney. The approach used depends on the pathology, lesion size, extent, required access, and surgeon preference. A transperitoneal or a retroperitoneoscopic approach may be used. Port placement depends on pathology, lesion size, extent, required access, and surgeon preference and requires 3–4 ports. Hand-assisted techniques are used in some centers. Laparoscopic nephrectomy has become the preferred technique for nephrectomy for benign indications in noninfected kidneys. Laparoscopic partial nephrectomy for small renal cell carcinoma (T1a, <4 cm in diameter) is preferred in some centers and has been shown to carry favorable oncological outcomes. In general, surgery is determined by the extent of disease with the laparoscopic approach confined to smaller tumors generally under 7 cm diameter, but larger tumors can be removed depending on the surgeons' experience and skill. Resection of the kidney, adrenal glands, and proximal ureter is usual, with surrounding lymph nodes, and involved organs, if appropriate. Removal of a surrounding bladder cuff around the vesicoureteric junction may be required. Hilar clamping and warm renal ischemia time remain a controversial issue in laparoscopic partial nephrectomy in view of the preservation of renal function (which is the underlying issue in partial nephrectomy). The port sites are usually closed deeply using absorbable muscle sutures and the skin closed with suture, staples, or tapes.

Anatomical Points

The kidneys develop as three successive sets of organs between the 4th and 8th week of gestation and migrate to about the L1 level by birth. Both kidneys may be joined anteriorly, forming a single horseshoe kidney, or each kidney may be segmented with separate ureteric drainage and/or vascular supply. Duplex ureteric systems are not uncommon. Ectopic kidneys or unilateral renal agenesis can occur. Congenital anomalies of the renal system may underlie vesicoureteric reflux or renal failure. The anatomical extent of the tumor determines the surgery required, and this may be planned preoperatively using ultrasound and CT or MRI.

Perspective

See Table 9.2. For small renal tumors, the procedure of laparoscopic nephrectomy or partial nephrectomy is relatively well defined and, overall, carries little risk. For more advanced tumors, an open procedure is preferable. With any laparoscopic surgery, the patient should be prewarned of the risk of conversion to an open procedure. Severe bleeding and injury to adjacent structures are the most immediate issues that can lead to further major complications, such as infection, peritonitis, and abscess formation. Injury to the pancreas, especially with left renal surgery, may invoke pancreatitis or pancreatic leakage. Seromas are not uncommon, while lymphatic

Table 9.2 Laparoscopic nephrectomy or laparoscopic partial nephrectomy estimated frequency of complications, risks, and consequences

Complications, risks, and consequences	Estimated frequency
Most significant/serious complications	
Infection[a]	
Subcutaneous/wound	1–5 %
Urinary/systemic	1–5 %
Intra-abdominal	1–5 %
Chest infection	1–5 %
Basal atelectasis	5–20 %
Bleeding/hematoma/seroma/lymphocele/lymph ascites/fistula[b]	1–5 %
Paralytic ileus[b]	1–5 %
Renal impairment	5–20 %
Urine leakage/urine collection (urinoma)[b]	5–20 %
Small bowel obstruction (early or late)[a]	1–5 %
Conversion to open operation	1–5 %
Rare significant/serious problems	
Pancreatitis/pancreatic injury/cyst/leakage/fistula	0.1–1 %
Diaphragmatic injury[a]	<0.1 %
Injury to the bowel or blood vessels (trochar or diathermy) [Duodenal/gastric/small bowel/colonic/iliac/mesenteric]	0.1–1 %
Bladder injury[a]	<0.1 %
Gas embolus	0.1–1 %
Pneumothorax	0.1–1 %
Deep venous thrombosis/pulmonary embolism	0.1–1 %
Splenectomy[c]	0.1–1 %
Multisystem organ failure[a]	0.1–1 %
Death[a]	<0.1 %
Less serious complications	
Pain/discomfort/tenderness	
Short term (<4 weeks)	1–5 %
Longer term (>12 weeks)	0.1–1 %
Urinary retention/catheterization	0.1–1 %
Nerve injury/sensory changes (lumbar plexus/branches, sympathetic chain)[a]	0.1–1 %
Wound scarring (deformity/dimpling of wound scar/poor cosmesis)	0.1–1 %
Port-site hernia (avoid lifting/straining for 8 weeks)	0.1–1 %
Drain tube(s)[a]	5–20 %

[a]Dependent on underlying pathology, surgical technique preferences, and location on the body
[b]Incidence may be higher for large or extensive masses
[c]Splenic preservation may sometimes be possible for splenic traumatic injury

collections are rare. Both may not be symptomatic, unless they become large, compress other structures, or become infected. Small bowel obstruction due to adhesions can occur after transperitoneal laparoscopic procedures. The aim of partial nephrectomy is to preserve some renal function. A critical issue in partial nephrectomy remains hilar clamping as renal cooling is technically not feasible (unlike in open partial nephrectomy) and warm ischemia times of more than 30 min are detrimental for renal function.

Major Complications/Consequences

Bleeding is one of the major potential complications of nephrectomy. **Transfusion** is rarely required. Slow ooze and either **seroma** or **hematoma formation** can occur, and **secondary infection** may develop sometimes leading to **abscess formation**. **Specific complications of partial nephrectomy** are urinary bleeding (**macroscopic hematuria**) and/or **urine extravasation**. Both may successfully be treated conservatively and may require endoscopic ureteric stenting, endovascular embolization, or open revision. **Peritonitis** can also be a significant complication. **Port-site hernia formation** can occur. Infection may occasionally lead to **systemic sepsis** and even **multisystem organ failure**, which is a significant cause of early **mortality** when it occurs. Later mortality is due to **tumor recurrence or persistence**. **Pancreatic leak**, collection, and **fistula** are very rare. **Gas embolism**, **major vascular injury**, or **bowel injury** are relatively rare. **Bowel injury** may very rarely require **stoma formation**. Splenic injury and **splenectomy** are rare complications with laparoscopic left nephrectomy. Significant **lymphatic leakage** may occur from **thoracic duct injury**, leading to **lymphatic ascites or collection**. **Small bowel obstruction** may be a recurrent major issue after transperitoneal laparoscopic renal surgery, often treated well conservatively, but surgery may be required.

Consent and Risk Reduction

Main Points to Explain

- GA risk
- Bleeding/hematoma
- Infection (local/systemic)
- Respiratory complications
- Deep venous thrombosis/pulmonary embolism
- Renal impairment
- Urine leakage/urine collection*
- Other abdominal organ injury
- Pain/discomfort
- Possible tumor recurrence*
- Possible blood transfusion
- Possible open surgery (if laparoscopic)
- Risks without surgery

*Dependent on pathology and type of surgery performed

Further Reading, References, and Resources

Nephrectomy or Partial Nephrectomy

Arancibia MF, Bolenz C, Michel MS, Keeley Jr FX, Alken P. The modern management of upper tract urothelial cancer: surgical treatment. BJU Int. 2007;99(5):978–81.

Dave DS, Lam JS, Leppert JT, Belldegrun AS. Open surgical management of renal cell carcinoma in the era of minimally invasive kidney surgery. BJU Int. 2005;96(9):1268–74.

Jamieson GG. The anatomy of general surgical operations. 2nd ed. Edinburgh: Churchill Livingston; 2006.

Joudi FN, Allareddy V, et al. Analysis of complications following partial and total nephrectomy for renal cancer in a population based sample. J Urol. 2007;177:1709–14.

Karakiewicz PI, Hutterer GC. Predicting cancer-control outcomes in patients with renal cell carcinoma. Curr Opin Urol. 2007;17(5):295–302.

McKiernan J, Simmons R, et al. Natural history of chronic renal insufficiency after partial and radical nephrectomy. Urology. 2002;59:816–20.

Neill MG, Jewett MA. The once and future role of cytoreductive nephrectomy. Urol Oncol. 2008;26(4):346–52.

Patard JJ, Shvarts O, Lam JS, et al. Safety and efficacy of partial nephrectomy for all T1 tumours based on an international multicenter experience. J Urol. 2004;171(6; 1):2181–5.

Shekarriz B, Upadhyay J, Shekarriz H, et al. Comparison of costs and complications of radical and partial nephrectomy for treatment of localized renal cell carcinoma. Urology. 2002;59:211–5.

Stephenson AJ, Hakimi AA, et al. Complications of radical and partial nephrectomy in a large contemporary cohort. J Urol. 2004;171:130–5.

Van Poppel H, Pozzo D, et al. A prospective randomized EORTC intergroup phase 3 study comparing the complications of elective nephron sparing surgery and radical nephrectomy for low-stage renal cell carcinoma. Eur Urol. 2007;51:1606–15.

Wszolek MF, Wotkowicz C, Libertino JA. Surgical management of large renal tumors. Nat Clin Pract Urol. 2008;5(1):35–46.

Laparoscopic Nephrectomy or Laparoscopic Partial Nephrectomy

Burgess NA, Koo BC, Calvert RC, et al. Randomized trial of laparoscopic v open nephrectomy. J Endourol. 2007;21:610–3.

Campbell SC, Novick AC. Expanding the indications for elective partial nephrectomy: is this advisable? Eur Urol. 2006;49(6):952–4.

Gill IS, Matin SF, Desai MM, et al. Comparative analysis of laparoscopic versus open partial nephrectomy for renal tumours in 200 patients. J Urol. 2003;170:64–8.

Jamieson GG. The anatomy of general surgical operations. 2nd ed. Edinburgh: Churchill Livingston; 2006.

Lesage K, Joniau S, Fransis K, Van Poppel H. Comparison between open partial and radical nephrectomy for renal tumours: perioperative outcome and health-related quality of life. Eur Urol. 2007;51(3):614–20.

Porpiglia F, Volpe A, Billia M, Scarpa RM. Laparoscopic versus open partial nephrectomy: analysis of the current literature. Eur Urol. 2008;53(4):732–42.

Shuford MD, McDougall EM, Chang SS, et al. Complications of contemporary radical nephrectomy : comparison of open vs laparoscopic approach. Urol Oncol. 2004;22:121–6.

Simforoosh N, Basiri A, et al. Comparison of laparoscopic and open donor nephrectomy; a randomized controlled trial. Br J Urol Int. 2005;95:851–5.

Simmons MN, Schreiber MJ, Gill IS. Surgical renal ischemia: a contemporary overview. J Urol. 2008;180(1):19–30.

Weise ES, Winfield HN. Laparoscopic partial nephrectomy. J Endourol. 2005;19(6):634–42.

Chapter 10
Renal Transplant Surgery

Christine Russell, Peter Morris, and Brendon J. Coventry

General Perspective and Overview

Renal transplantation covers a spectrum of donor, recipient, surgeon, and institutional variables, which often have a significant impact upon risks, complications, and outcomes. Allografts may come from cadaveric or live donors, and this alone can also determine the range and frequency of complications experienced. Recipient variables are broader and relate to the underlying disease process that has necessitated the renal transplantation. Failure of the grafted kidney can occur from continuation of the underlying disease process to affect the new kidney, which can subsequently lead to failure of the transplant.

Complications in renal transplantation can be broadly divided into early (intra-operative), intermediate (immediate or in-hospital postoperative), and late (delayed; post-discharge). Bleeding is usually controlled at surgery, but may necessitate blood transfusion or occasionally occur postoperatively, and rarely requires surgical evacuation of a hematoma. Bleeding tendency is another variable in this equation. Collection of lymph or leakage of urine can predispose to infection, which can lead to systemic sepsis and rarely to death. Urinary obstruction and infection are not uncommon sequelae. Longer-term problems with immunosuppressive therapy, including opportunistic infections and malignancy, can be serious, but this must be

---

C. Russell, BA, BM, BCh, FRACS (✉)
Central and Northern Adelaide Renal and Transplantation Service, Royal Adelaide Hospital,
Adelaide, Australia
e-mail: christine.russell3@health.sa.gov.au

P. Morris, AC FRS FMed Sci, FRCP, FRCS
University of Oxford, Oxford, UK

B.J. Coventry, BMBS, PhD, FRACS, FACS, FRSM
Discipline of Surgery, Royal Adelaide Hospital, University of Adelaide,
L5 Eleanor Harrald Building, North Terrace, 5000 Adelaide, SA, Australia
e-mail: brendon.coventry@adelaide.edu.au

B.J. Coventry (ed.), *Cardio-Thoracic, Vascular, Renal and Transplant Surgery*, 157
Surgery: Complications, Risks and Consequences,
DOI 10.1007/978-1-4471-5418-1_10, © Springer-Verlag London 2014

balanced against continued dialysis or death. If the grafted kidney fails, continued dialysis or re-transplantation will usually be required.

This chapter deals with the broad consideration of risks, complications, and consequences related to renal transplantation, and the relative frequencies must be modified for specific situations, patients, and comorbidities accordingly. Where the timing of a complication is not specifically mentioned, the estimated frequency represents figures for the overall relative risk of that complication.

With these factors and facts in mind, the information given in these chapters must be appropriately and discernibly interpreted and used.

The **use of specialized units with standardized preoperative assessment, multidisciplinary input, and high-quality postoperative care** is essential to the success of complex transplant surgery overall and can significantly reduce the risk of complications or aid early detection, prompt intervention, and cost.

The authors would like to thank Dr Mohan Rao, Adelaide, Australia, for his advice.

> **Important Note**
> It should be emphasized that the risks and frequencies that are given here *represent derived figures. These figures are best estimates of relative frequencies across most institutions*, not merely the highest-performing ones, and as such are often representative of a number of studies, which include different patients with differing comorbidities and different surgeons. In addition, the risks of complications in lower or higher risk patients may lie outside these estimated ranges, and individual clinical judgement is required as to the expected risks communicated to the patient, staff, or for other purposes. The range of risks is also derived from experience and the literature; while risks outside this range may exist, certain risks may be reduced or absent due to variations of procedures or surgical approaches. It is recognized that different patients, practitioners, institutions, regions, and countries may vary in their requirements and recommendations.

Renal Transplant (Allograft) Surgery

Description

General anesthesia is used, though the procedure can be performed under epidural or spinal anesthesia if required. The aim of the procedure is to graft an allogeneic kidney into a patient with renal failure to restore renal function. An oblique incision is made in the lateral lower abdomen at the level and in front of the anterior superior iliac spine. The muscles of the abdominal wall are cut and separated in layers. The bladder is filled at the start of the operation to make its identification easier. An extraperitoneal plane is developed in the iliac fossa. The kidney is then dissected with great care to avoid damaging small vessels, in particular accessory arteries. The renal vessels are sutured to the external iliac vessels; occasionally the artery is joined to the internal iliac if there is no aortic patch. Bleeding can occur at clamp release, occasionally requiring reclamping. The ureter is sutured to the bladder with an attempt at an anti-reflux mechanism. The kidney must be placed to avoid any kinking of the vessels. Placement of a drain depends on individual preference. A mass or muscle layer closure is made, and an interrupted subcutaneous absorbable suture with a continuous subcuticular suture or staples is used.

Anatomical Points

The external iliac vein is deeper on the left. The kidney may have two or more vessels (15 % have multiple renal arteries). Smaller renal veins can be ligated. Renal arteries are best left on the donor aortic patch. If using a live donor, there is no aortic patch and the renal artery can be anastomosed end to end to the internal iliac artery. A duplex ureteric system may also be present.

Perspective

See Table 10.1. Thrombosis of the vessels is rare, about 1 % in most series, but is obviously of great consequence to the patient, as the kidney is usually lost. Care must be taken with vascular suturing and also with placement of the kidney to avoid kinking or stretching of the vessels. The positioning of the kidney can be difficult, especially with the right kidney as the artery is substantially longer than the vein and may have a tendency to kink. Care must be taken to ligate lymphatic vessels, both around the iliac vessels and the renal artery, to diminish the risk of lymphocele formation. Collections are relatively common, up to 50 % in some series, but most are small and resolve spontaneously. Only those causing problems such as pressure on the ureter or vascular structures require further intervention. Necrosis or stricturing of the ureter requires a longer stay in hospital and further surgery, but is not usually of any long-term consequence. It is important to distend the bladder to avoid inadvertently suturing the ureter to the peritoneum. The operation is extraperitoneal (except in small children), so intraperitoneal complications such as paralytic ileus are uncommon. Wound infections can be severe, with the kidney exposed in some cases. These open wounds may take months to heal, because of the immunosuppression. Infection around the vessels can lead to anastomotic infection and life-threatening hemorrhage. This is fortunately extremely rare.

Table 10.1 Renal transplantation estimated frequency of complications, risks, and consequences

Complications, risks, and consequences	Estimated frequency
Most significant/serious complications	
Infection (overall)	20–50 %
Wound	1–5 %
Urinary	20–50 %
Central nervous system	0.1–1 %
Systemic	1–5 %
Opportunistic (CMV[a], candidiasis, pneumocystis)	20–50 %
Gastrointestinal erosion, ulceration, perforation	5–20 %
Abnormal LFTs	5–20 %
Bleeding or hematoma formation	
Wound	1–5 %
Perigraft	1–5 %
Paralytic ileus	1–5 %
Significant lymphocele/seroma formation	1–5 %
Ureteric ischemia (causing leak or obstruction)	1–5 %
Vesicoureteric reflux (depends on method of reimplantation)	5–20 %
Thrombosis	
Renal artery	0.1–1 %
Renal vein	1–5 %
Renal transplant arterial stenosis – late	1–5 %
Allograft rejection (overall)	20–50 %
Early/late acute (dependant on immunosuppression used)	20–50 %
Chronic	20–50 %
Hyperacute (very rare with current crossmatch techniques)	<0.1 %
Delayed graft function	5–20 %
Immunosuppression toxicity (nephro-/neuro-/myelotoxicity)	20–50 %
Neural injury [e.g., lateral cutaneous nerve of thigh, compressed by retractors]	1–5 %
Malignancy (long term)	20–50 %
Skin malignancy (long term)[b]	20–50 %
Non-skin malignancy (long term)	5–20 %
Rare significant/serious problems	
Cerebral ischemia/hemorrhage/thrombosis (CVA; TIA; RIND)[c]	0.1–1 %
Deep venous thrombosis/pulmonary embolus	0.1–1 %
Pancreatitis	0.1–1 %
Multisystem organ failure[c]	0.1–1 %
Death (<30 days)[c]	0.1–1 %
Less serious complications	
Pain/tenderness [wound pain]	
Acute (<4 weeks)	>80 %
Chronic (>12 weeks)	1–5 %
Incisional hernia formation (delayed heavy lifting or straining)	1–5 %
Wound scarring/deformity – poor cosmesis	1–5 %
Blood transfusion[c]	1–5 %
Wound drain[c]	Individual

Complications, risks, and consequences	Estimated frequency
Ancillary medical complications	
Posttransplant diabetes	5–20 %
Hyperlipidemia	20–50 %
Hypertension	50–80 %
Cardiovascular disease	50–80 %
Cataracts	50–80 %
Bone osteodystrophy	20–50 %
Polycythemia	5–20 %

[a]NB: CMV infection depends on the unit's policy on transplantation of CMV + ve donor grafts into CMV−ve recipients
[b]Dependent on latitude and UV exposure (i.e., 50 % at 20 years in Australia)
[c]Dependent on underlying pathology, anatomy, surgical technique, and surgeon preferences

Major Complications

Technical complications are related to the two main parts of the operation – **vascular** and **urological**. The renal vessels are sutured to the external iliac vessels and the kidney is placed in an extraperitoneal pocket. **Bleeding** can occur, but rarely necessitates a return to theatre. (NB: uremic platelets are not as sticky as normal ones so bleeding tendency is higher.) **Thrombosis** can also occur, either of the artery or vein, which usually results **renal necrosis**, necessitating **kidney loss and removal**. Rarely, an incomplete occlusion of the vein can be remedied with rescue of the graft. It is important to place the kidney in such a position that the vessels are not compromised. Urological complications are relatively common. The blood supply of the transplanted ureter must all come from the renal artery and this may be inadequate. This has two consequences – either **necrosis of the distal ureter** with the development of a **urine leak** or **ureteric stricture** formation, leading to **hydronephrosis** and **impaired renal function**. These two problems can usually be rectified, either by a direct reimplantation, with or without a psoas hitch, or implantation into a Boari flap. Anastomosis of the transplanted ureter to the native ureter is also sometimes undertaken. **Lymph collections** can occur around the kidney. The risk of this can be diminished with care to ligate small lymphatic vessels around the iliac vessels and also around the renal artery. **Collections of pus**, **serum**, or **urine** may also develop. Asymptomatic lymphoceles can be left; those causing discomfort or compression of vessels or collecting system should be dealt with. This can be done initially by drainage with or without sclerosant, but may require de-roofing into the peritoneal cavity.

Longer-term complications include:

- **Infection**, particularly viral such as CMV.
- **Malignancy**, particularly squamous cell carcinoma of skin and lymphoma, for which the risk is about 1 %. Lymphoma is often related to EBV infection.

- **Chronic rejection** leading to graft loss.
- **Cardiovascular disease**.
- **Recurrent disease** affecting the new kidney, depending on the original disease.

Graft survival is:

1 year: 90 %
5 years: 79 %
10 years: 50 %

Patient survival is:

1 year: 95 %
5 years: 85 %
10 years: 70 %

Consent and Risk Reduction

Main Points to Explain

- GA risk
- Bleeding
- Wound infection
- Abscess formation
- Urinary problems
- Transplant failure
- Immunosuppressive therapy
- Malignancy
- Further surgery
- Risks without surgery

Further Reading, References, and Resources

Courtney AE, McNamee PT, Maxwell AP. The evolution of renal transplantation in clinical practice: for better, for worse? QJM. 2008;101(12):967–78.

de Souza RM, Olsburgh J. Urinary tract infection in the renal transplant patient. Nat Clin Pract Nephrol. 2008;4(5):252–64.

Morris PJ, editor. Kidney transplantation – principles and practices. 5th ed. Philadelphia: W.B.Saunders; 2001.

Nicol D, Hirst G. Urological assessment and complications in renal transplantation. Transplant Rev. 1999;13:12–22.

Säemann M, Hörl WH. Urinary tract infection in renal transplant recipients. Eur J Clin Invest. 2008;38 Suppl 2:58–65.

Chapter 11
Liver Transplant Surgery

Jonathon Fawcett, John Chen, and Brendon J. Coventry

General Perspective and Overview

Liver transplantation is reserved for selected patients with decompensated liver disease, where life expectancy is estimated to be less than 12 months or in patients with hepatocellular cancer and chronic liver disease where resection may not be tolerated. Occasionally, liver transplantation is undertaken for other malignancies, such as highly selected patients with cholangiocarcinoma, and also occasionally for metabolic disease with extrahepatic manifestations such as urea cycle disorders in infants. The numerous risks and potential complications associated with liver transplantation need to be balanced against the prospect of best supportive treatment (which often advances inexorably to death). The timing of transplantation is therefore a significant factor for each individual patient and situation but is also determined by donor organ availability. Overall, many of the relative risks and complications have progressively decreased over the last 25 years.

With these factors in mind, this chapter addresses some of the known and estimated risks associated with liver transplantation. The exact frequency of any

J. Fawcett, D. Phil, FRCS, FRACS (✉)
Queensland Liver Transplant Service, Princess Alexandra Hospital, Brisbane, Australia
e-mail: j.fawcett@uq.edu.au

J. Chen, MBBS, Ph.D., FRACS
South Australian Liver Transplant Unit, Flinders Medical Centre, Adelaide, Australia

B.J. Coventry, BMBS, PhD, FRACS, FACS, FRSM
Discipline of Surgery, Royal Adelaide Hospital, University of Adelaide,
L5 Eleanor Harrald Building, North Terrace, 5000 Adelaide, SA, Australia
e-mail: brendon.coventry@adelaide.edu.au

B.J. Coventry (ed.), *Cardio-Thoracic, Vascular, Renal and Transplant Surgery*,
Surgery: Complications, Risks and Consequences,
DOI 10.1007/978-1-4471-5418-1_11, © Springer-Verlag London 2014

complication and its relative risk represents a distinctly individual entity for many surgical procedures, and this point is significant when considering the inherent complexity of liver transplantation, which can magnify many of these risks.

As can be appreciated by the frequency table, the possible complications and consequences are myriad, but many of these can be prevented to reduce the attendant risks of these developing. Patient selection, as with many surgical procedures and many therapies, is paramount in controlling the risks associated with liver transplantation. The experience of the staff and the quality of the postoperative care are also substantial in determining the outcomes in many cases.

The initial disease for which the liver transplantation is being performed, and its extent, also has a significant bearing on the range and frequency of complications and consequences that are likely to be associated with a particular type of transplant in a particular patient.

Awareness of many of the potential complications can allow early diagnosis, intervention, treatment, and possible prevention. Some complications can be reversed or minimized. Complications in the perioperative and early postoperative period significantly contribute to early graft loss and death, while later deaths are usually attributable to complications of chronic immunosuppression, malignancy, cardiovascular events and cirrhosis, often from recrudescence of causative factors (e.g., alcohol and viral infections). Graft survival at 1 year is about 80 % and patient survival is around 85 %, reflecting the fact that some patients are transplanted more than once. For those patients successfully grafted with survival beyond 1 year, continued long-term survival is usual. However, in the short term, primary nonfunction of the liver, severe coagulopathy, renal failure, systemic infection, multisystem organ failure, air embolism, and acute rejection remain serious and significant problems. In the longer term, chronic rejection, chronic renal failure, recurrent liver disease (viral, autoimmune, and alcoholic), and cirrhosis also create significant causes of morbidity and mortality.

This chapter therefore attempts to draw together in one place the estimated overall frequencies of the complications associated with liver transplantation, based on information obtained from the literature and experience. Not all patients are at risk of the full range of listed complications. It must be individualized for each patient and their disease process, but represents a guide and summary of the attendant risks, complications, and consequences.

With these factors and facts in mind, the information given in this chapter must be appropriately and discernibly interpreted and used.

The **use of specialized units with standardized preoperative assessment, multidisciplinary input, and high-quality postoperative care** is essential to the success of complex liver transplantation surgery overall and significantly reduces risk of complications or aids early detection, prompt intervention, and cost.

Important Note

It should be emphasized that the risks and frequencies that are given here *represent derived figures. These figures are best estimates of relative frequencies across most institutions*, not merely the highest-performing ones, and as such are often representative of a number of studies, which include different patients with differing comorbidities and different surgeons. In addition, the risks of complications in lower or higher risk patients may lie outside these estimated ranges, and individual clinical judgement is required as to the expected risks communicated to the patient, staff, or for other purposes. The range of risks is also derived from experience and the literature; while risks outside this range may exist, certain risks may be reduced or absent due to variations of procedures or surgical approaches. It is recognized that different patients, practitioners, institutions, regions, and countries may vary in their requirements and recommendations.

For complications related to other associated/additional surgery that may arise during liver transplantation, see the relevant chapter, for example, small bowel surgery (volume 4) or thoracotomy (Chap. 7).

The authors would like to thank Professor Peter Friend, Oxford, UK, and Professor John McCall, Dunedin, NZ, for their helpful discussion and advice.

Liver Transplant Surgery

Description

General anesthesia is used. Liver transplantation is used for end-stage liver failure arising from a variety of causes, including highly selected patients with malignancy in the setting of liver disease. The procedure is invariably performed within a specialized unit with a team of hepatologists, anesthetists, nurses, intensivists, and surgeons. The aim is to graft an allogeneic liver into a patient with end-stage liver failure to restore liver function. Several variations in technique are described; however, the general principle is to anastomose the donor vena cava with the recipient cava, either end to end or end to side (the "piggyback" technique), and to restore continuity to the portal vein, hepatic artery, and common bile duct. Historically, whole livers from cadaveric donors have been used, but subsequent development has included "cutdown" or split livers (right and left sided grafts), initially to develop a source of transplant livers for children, but also to address donor shortage so that maximum use can be made of donor livers. For the same reason, living donor liver transplantation is now widely practiced worldwide. HLA matching does not reduce rejection rates in liver transplantation and would be logistically difficult within the time constraints of liver preservation.

Anatomical Points

The hepatic artery, portal vein, and bile duct are divided into a right and left trunk at the hilum of the liver. This division forms the two functional hemi-livers, which meet at the main fissure (hence the feasibility of split liver transplants). The right portal pedicle will either enter the liver or divide prior to entering the liver into a posterior and anterior sectorial branch, which supplies segments 6 and 7 and 5 and 8, respectively. Anastomoses are to the vena cava, hepatic artery, common bile duct, and portal vein. The attachments of the liver must be divided to properly mobilize the nonfunctioning liver for removal, and the donor liver occupies a similar position (orthotopic transplantation).

Perspective

See Table 11.1. Any consideration of complications in liver transplantation needs to be balanced against the risk in not performing the transplant, which is often death. The range and potential severity of complications associated with liver transplantation is considerable, due partly to the complexity of the procedure itself and the individual nature of the disease affecting the liver. Patient survival at 1 year is 85–95 % across most continents. Gradual gains have been made almost every year; however, continued gains in patient survival have reduced in the last few years, possibly because of broadened indications with expansion of criteria for liver transplantation, the transplantation of marginal recipients, and technical refinements have been essentially maximized, and because of the increasing use of marginal donor organs. In many centers, the most common causes of graft loss and patient death remain recurrent disease and de novo malignancies.

Early Complications

These include **primary graft nonfunction** (~1 % requiring urgent re-transplantation), **initial poor graft function** (~5 % – the increasing use of marginal cadaveric grafts increases the likelihood of poor graft function – an example of a marginal graft would be a donor liver with more than 30 % steatosis, especially if of macrovesicular distribution), and **postoperative bleeding** – liver transplantation is a major

Table 11.1 Liver transplant surgery estimated frequency of complications, risks, and consequences

Complications, risks, and consequences	Estimated frequency
Most significant/serious complications	
Early complications (≤90 days after surgery)	
Infection[a]	
Wound	5–20 %
Intra-abdominal (including liver subphrenic abscess)	1–5 %
Intrathoracic (pneumonia; pleural, mediastinitis)	20–50 %
Systemic	1–5 %
Opportunistic (CMV, candidiasis, pneumocystis)[a]	50–80 %
Vascular/coagulation related[a]	
Bleeding and hematoma overall	20–50 %
Arterial, venous (caval, renal, portal, hepatic, or lobar vessels)	5–20 %
Raw liver surface	5–20 %
Extrahepatic	
Chance of returning to the operating theatre for post-op bleeding	5–20 %
Vascular occlusion (all causes) (Non-thrombotic; partial or complete kinking; arterial stenosis)	5–20 %
Thrombosis	
Hepatic arterial	1–5 %
Portal venous	1–5 %
Hepatic venous	0.1–1 %
IVC complications (stenosis; kinking)[a]	1–5 %
Coagulopathy (all causes)	20–50 %
Disseminated intravascular coagulopathy	0.1–1 %
Consumption posttransfusion (large bleed)[a]	1–5 %
Deep venous thrombosis	0.1–1 %
Liver related[a]	
Subcapsular liver hematoma[a] (major, at transplantation or liver biopsy)	5–20 %
Hepatitis (drug, CMV, recurrent)[a]	5–20 %
Primary liver transplant nonfunction[a]	2–5 %
Common/extrahepatic/intrahepatic bile duct injury	1–5 %
Bile collections	1–5 %
Budd-Chiari (acute)[a]	0.1–1 %
GI related[a]	
Seroma/lymphocele formation[a]	20–50 %
Gastrointestinal injury, erosion, ulceration, perforation, hemorrhage	5–20 %
Pancreatic or duodenal injury/fistula/pancreatitis	1–5 %
Small bowel obstruction (early or late)[a] [Ischemic stenosis/adhesion formation]	1–5 %
Possibility of colostomy/ileostomy (very rare)[a]	<0.1 %
Splenic injury	0.1–1 %
Conservation (consequent limitation to activity; late rupture)	
Splenectomy	
Lung/chest related[a]	
Pneumothorax or pulmonary injury (direct)	50–80 %
Pleural effusions[a]	20–50 %

(continued)

Table 11.1 (continued)

Complications, risks, and consequences	Estimated frequency
Chest infection[a]	5–20 %
Surgical emphysema[a](major)	1–5 %
Thoracic duct injury (chylous leak, fistula)[a]	1–5 %
Aspiration pneumonitis	0.1–1 %
Air embolus (major)	0.1–1 %
Diaphragmatic injury hernia or paresis	0.1–1 %
Cardiac related[a]	
Cardiac arrhythmias (major)	20–50 %
Pericardial effusion	1–5 %
Myocardial injury/cardiac failure infarction (hypotension)	1–5 %
Renal related	
Acute renal failure (including hepatorenal syndrome)	5–20 %
Renal/adrenal injury renal vein[a]	1–5 %
Metabolic	
Hypoglycemia	5–20 %
Hyperglycemia	1–5 %
Neurological	
Sleep disturbance, mental disturbance	50–80 %
Seizures	1–5 %
Cerebral edema	1–5 %
Wound dehiscence[a]	0.1–1 %
Multisystem organ failure (renal, pulmonary, cardiac failure)[a]	1–5 %
Early mortality[a]	5–20 %
Intermediate complications (90–360 days after surgery)	
Biliary related and fluid leaks[a]	
Hyperbilirubinemia	50–80 %
Biliary and serous/lymph ascites	20–50 %
Bile duct obstruction (any cause) [Ischemia; stenosis]	5–20 %
Bile leak	5–20 %
Biliary collection	5–20 %
Biliary fistula	1–5 %
Persistent clinical jaundice	1–5 %
Rejection[a]	
Early/late acute/hyperacute	20–50 %
Chronic	0.1–1 %
Late complications (≥360 days after surgery)	
Chronic liver rejection[a]	5–20 %
Neurological[a](peripheral and central nervous systems)	5–20 %
Chronic renal failure (5–10 years)[a]	20–50 %
Immunosuppression toxicity[a]	5–20 %
Posttransplant malignancies (long term)[a]	
Skin cancers (long term)[a]	>80 %
Lymphoproliferative disorders (lymphoma)[a]	5–20 %
Carcinomas[a]	Individual
Recurrence of malignancy (if transplanted for malignancy)[a]	Individual

Table 11.1 (continued)

Complications, risks, and consequences	Estimated frequency
Recurrent cirrhosis (all causes)[a] [Hep B, C, alcohol, biliary cirrhosis, sclerosing cholangitis, autoimmune hepatitis]	20–50 %
Biliary[a](all causes: stones, stenosis, recurrent cholangitis, sclerosis)	5–20 %
Metabolic	
Hyperlipidemia	20–50 %
Hyperglycemia	5–20 %
Osteoporosis	5–20 %
Graft-versus-host disease (GVHD)[a]	0.1–1 %
Graft loss[a]	
1 year (~10 %)[b]	5–20 %
5 year (~25 %)[b]	20–50 %
Late mortality[a]	5–20 %
Less serious complications	
Pain/tenderness [rib pain (sternal retractor), wound pain]	
Acute (<4 weeks)	>80 %
Chronic (>12 weeks)[a]	5–20 %
Paralytic ileus	20–50 %
Reflux esophagitis/pharyngitis/pneumonitis	1–5 %
Delayed gastric emptying	20–50 %
Nutritional deficiency – anemia, B12 malabsorption[a]	5–20 %
Wound scarring (poor cosmesis/wound deformity)	5–20 %
Incisional hernia formation (delayed heavy lifting/straining for 8–12 weeks)[a]	1–5 %
Nasogastric tube[a]	1–5 %
Blood transfusion[a]	5–20 %
Wound drain tube(s)[a]	50–80 %

[a]Dependent on the underlying pathology, anatomy, surgical technique, preferences, and comorbidities; the risks represent estimated ranges for the spectrum of frequency associated with the respective complication. Some cases may lie outside these predicted ranges depending on the situation
[b]Australian New Zealand liver transplant 1-year patient survival is approximately 90 % and 80 % at 5 years over the last 20 years. Patient survival had continued to improve over the last 25 years in all jurisdictions

operation often undertaken in the setting of thrombocytopenia, severe coagulopathy, and portal hypertension. Thus, there is a 10 % or more chance of such patients needing reexploration for postoperative hemorrhage. Usually, this will be from the surgical field, but can be from other sites, e.g., rarely, cirrhotic patients develop splenic artery aneurysms that can rupture early after transplant. **Hepatic arterial thrombosis (HAT)** – in about 2–5 % of cases (higher incidence in children) – the outcome of arterial thrombosis ranges from catastrophic liver failure through biliary necrosis to multiple hepatic abscesses, but occasionally the graft continues to function normally (the propensity for biliary complications relates to the near absolute dependence of bile ducts on an arterial blood supply, while hepatocytes can maintain viability with a portal supply alone). Roughly though, HAT results in a 1 in 3 chance of needing re-transplantation. HAT occasionally presents years after transplantation, sometimes manifesting as a pyogenic liver abscess – and is less likely then to result in graft loss.

Portal vein thrombosis – while it may result in continuing portal hypertension – does not often threaten the graft. Thrombectomy does not reliably reestablish vein patency. **Hepatic vein thrombosis** is virtually unheard of, but stenosis manifests in the early postoperative period as ascites, and a technical problem with the "top" venous anastomosis may cause severe intraoperative congestion of the liver – this is a rare, but fearsome, intraoperative situation to deal with. **Acute rejection** occurs in 30–40 % of patients depending on the immunosuppressive regimen used and is virtually always straightforward to treat with pulse steroids. Monoclonal antibody therapy against T cells is not often needed in liver transplantation – acute rejection is generally much less of a problem compared to other areas of solid organ transplantation. **Infection** – CMV infection or reactivation peaking at 6 weeks posttransplant – is almost the norm in liver transplant patients especially in CMV-naïve recipients of CMV-positive grafts and is usually easily treated with antiviral therapy (ganciclovir). Different infections tend to occur at typical time points after transplantation, thus CMV infection peaks at 6 weeks postoperatively, but toxoplasmosis and nocardia infection occur at later time points. Most transplant recipients are usually not troubled by serious infection; nonetheless, specialist units regularly see transplant patients with either common organisms manifesting with unusual patterns of infection or unusual organisms giving rise to infection – an example of the latter would be mucormycosis of the paranasal sinuses, a devastating disease that frequently pursues an indolent, but fatal course. The rule in the immunosuppressed patient is to "expect the unexpected". **Postoperative ascites** (25 %), **pleural effusions** (50 %), **subphrenic abscess** (5 %), and **bile collections** (5 %). Patients with preoperative ascites or hydrothorax often develop the same fluid accumulation up to 3 months after transplant. Pleural effusion is common in all groups of recipients and reflects the magnitude of the surgery below the diaphragm. Postoperative infective collections, typically in the subphrenic spaces (sometimes the pelvis), also occur, more commonly after split or cutdown livers are transplanted (the "raw" surface may leak bile or blood and can then become infected). **Biliary complications** (~15 %) – 1 in 6 patients develop a biliary complication, either a bile leak leading to a postoperative collection or frank peritonitis or, alternatively, a biliary anastomotic stricture. Strictures can present at any time after transplant, but most commonly in the first 3 months. Some centers consider split grafts are more prone to biliary complications, and the early era of living-related liver transplants in adults (which utilized a right hemi-graft) was beset with biliary sequelae.

Late Complications

Graft loss – about 10 % at 1 year and 25 % at 5 years – occurs either because the graft fails due to chronic rejection, as the end point of an anastomotic problem (**hepatic arterial thrombosis** or occasionally **unreconstructable biliary stricturing**), or because the original liver disease recurs in the graft and finally if the patient dies for any other reason (such as recurrence of malignancy, if this was the indication for transplantation). **Recurrence of the original liver disease** varies from 0 % (for reformed alcoholics) through 25 % (primary biliary cirrhosis, primary sclerosing cholangitis) to nearly 100 % (hepatitis C infection). Hepatitis C reinfection, while nearly universal, unpredictably results in graft damage, but cirrhosis may recur in up to 25 %, and antiviral therapy, so far, has not been very successful. Re-transplantation is the solution to graft failure, but sometimes results in a more accelerated course to graft failure in the 2nd transplant. **Chronic renal failure or impairment** (~30 %), **accelerated cardiovascular disease, and osteoporosis**. Most of the other long-term sequelae of liver transplantation relate to immunosuppression. The introduction of the calcineurin antagonists, cyclosporine A, and (later) tacrolimus, revolutionized outcomes in solid organ transplantation, but the main long-term drawback has been renal toxicity. The keys to reducing the toxicity of immunosuppression has been to use drugs in combination, permitting lower individual doses and tapering immunosuppression dosing after transplantation to the lowest levels commensurate with prevention of rejection. Liver transplants have the lowest rates of rejection of all solid organ transplants and long-term; only very low levels of immunosuppression are needed. **Malignancy** (100 %) – if liver transplant patients live long enough, eventually all will get at least one skin cancer and some patients become afflicted with dozens of nonmelanoma skin cancers every year. Solid organ cancers otherwise occur at much the same rate as the general population. However, a specific malignancy that can occur in all transplant recipients is posttransplant lymphoproliferative disorder (PTLD) – this is an EBV-driven B-cell lymphoma. This is most common in children, because they are more frequently EBV naïve, and also in those patients who have required a lot of immunosuppression such as those needing pulse steroids or, especially, anti-T-cell antibody treatment for acute rejection. Patients with HCC who receive a transplant are at risk of tumor recurrence, although this is uncommon (<10 %) if only patients with early stage tumors are transplanted, but while rarely done, transplantation for cholangiocarcinoma is frequently associated with tumor recurrence (50 % or more).

Major Complications

Awareness of many of the potential complications can allow early diagnosis, intervention, treatment, and possible prevention. Some complications can be reversed or minimized. Although there are a number of severe complications, which may lead to mortality, it is important to recognize that without surgery, early mortality would be certain in almost all cases. Short-term major complications include **bleeding**, which may necessitate **return to theatre, primary nonfunction of the liver, severe coagulopathy, acute renal failure, systemic infection, multisystem organ failure, air embolism,** and **acute rejection,** which can be serious and significant, with high risk of **death.** Longer-term major complications including **chronic rejection, chronic renal failure, recurrent liver disease (viral, autoimmune, and alcoholic)** and **cirrhosis** also create significant causes of morbidity and mortality. **Hernia formation** is relatively common due to the large incision dividing abdominal wall muscles and nerves. The risk of **malignancy** increases with prolonged immunosuppressive therapy, although most of this excess risk is for skin cancers.

Consent and Risk Reduction

Main Points to Explain

- GA risk
- Major bleeding
- Wound infection
- Liver rejection/failure
- Multiorgan failure
- Bowel injury/perforation
- Peritonitis/abscess formation
- Malignancy
- Delayed mobilization/lifting/straining
- Death
- Risks without surgery

Further Reading, References, and Resources

Aguilera V, Berenguer M, Rubín A, San-Juan F, Rayón JM, Prieto M, Mir J. Cirrhosis of mixed etiology (hepatitis C virus and alcohol): posttransplantation outcome-comparison with hepatitis C virus-related cirrhosis and alcoholic-related cirrhosis. Liver Transpl. 2009;15(1): 79–87.

Appleton CP, Hurst RT. Reducing coronary artery disease events in liver transplant patients: moving toward identifying the vulnerable patient. Liver Transpl. 2008;14(12):1691–3.

Belongia EA, Costa J, Gareen IF, Grem JL, Inadomi JM, Kern ER, McHugh JA, Petersen GM, Rein MF, Sorrell MF, Strader DB, Trotter HT. NIH consensus development statement on management of hepatitis B. NIH Consens State Sci Statements. 2008;25(2):1–29.

Bindi ML, Biancofiore G, Esposito M, Meacci L, Bisà M, Mozzo R, Urbani L, Catalano G, Montin U, Filipponi F. Transcranial doppler sonography is useful for the decision-making at the point of care in patients with acute hepatic failure: a single centre's experience. J Clin Monit Comput. 2008;22(6):449–52.

Burgos L, Hernández F, Barrena S, Andres AM, Encinas JL, Leal N, Gamez M, Murcia J, Jara P, Lopez-Santamaria M, Tovar JA. Variant techniques for liver transplantation in pediatric programs. Eur J Pediatr Surg. 2008;18(6):372–4.

Chamlian V, Cherid A, Cherid N, Boutaghou HO, Chamlian A. Prognosis of human liver transplantation. Cell Mol Biol (Noisy-le-grand). 2008;54(Suppl):OL1062–76.

de Rougemont O, Dutkowski P, Weber M, Clavien PA. Abdominal drains in liver transplantation: useful tool or useless dogma? A matched case–control study. Liver Transpl. 2009;15(1): 96–101.

Deberaldini M, Arcanjo AB, Melo E, da Silva RF, Felício HC, Arroyo Jr PC, Duca WJ, Cordeiro JA, da Silva RC. Hepatopulmonary syndrome: morbidity and survival after liver transplantation. Transplant Proc. 2008;40(10):3512–6.

Della Rocca G, Costa MG, Pompei L, Chiarandini P. The liver transplant recipient with cardiac disease. Transplant Proc. 2008;40(4):1172–4.

Karasu Z, Akyildiz M, Kilic M, Zeytunlu M, Aydin U, Tekin F, Yilmaz F, Ozacar T, Akarca U, Ersoz G, Gunsar F, Ilter T, Lucey MR. Living donor liver transplantation for hepatitis B cirrhosis. J Gastroenterol Hepatol. 2007;22(12):2124–9.

Kilic M, Aydin U, Noyan A, Arikan C, Aydogdu S, Akyildiz M, Karasu Z, Zeytunlu M, Alper M, Batur Y. Live donor liver transplantation for acute liver failure. Transplantation. 2007;84(4):475–9.

Kim BW, Park YK, Kim YB, Wang HJ, Kim MW. Salvage liver transplantation for recurrent hepatocellular carcinoma after liver resection: feasibility of the milan criteria and operative risk. Transplant Proc. 2008;40(10):3558–61.

Lang H, Sotiropoulos GC, Beckebaum S, Fouzas I, Molmenti EP, Omar OS, Sgourakis G, Radtke A, Nadalin S, Saner FH, Malagó M, Gerken G, Paul A, Broelsch CE. Incidence of liver retransplantation and its effect on patient survival. Transplant Proc. 2008;40(9):3201–3.

Ling L, He X, Zeng J, Liang Z. In-hospital cerebrovascular complications following orthotopic liver transplantation: a retrospective study. BMC Neurol. 2008;8(1):52.

Meneu-Diaz JC, Moreno-Gonzalez E, Garcia I, Moreno-Elola A, Perez Saborido B, Fundora Suarez Y, Jimenez-Galanes S, Olivares S, Hidalgo Pascual M, Abradelo M, Jimenez C. Starting a new program of split liver transplantation after a low learning curve: a reality in centers with large experience in liver surgery and whole liver transplantation. Hepatogastroenterology. 2008;55(86–87):1699–704.

Mercado MA, Vilatobá M, Chan C, Domínguez I, Leal RP, Olivera MA. Intrahepatic bilioenteric anastomosis after biliary complications of liver transplantation: operative rescue of surgical failures. World J Surg. 2009;33(3):534–8.

Muscari F, Guinard JP, Foppa B, Trocard P, Danjoux M, Kamel MS, Duffas JP, Rostaing L, Fourtanier G, Suc B. Biological changes after liver transplantation according to the presence or not of graft steatosis. Transplant Proc. 2008;40(10):3562–5.

Ng VL, Fecteau A, Shepherd R, Magee J, Bucuvalas J, Alonso E, McDiarmid S, Cohen G, Anand R, Studies of Pediatric Liver Transplantation Research Group. Outcomes of 5-year survivors of pediatric liver transplantation: report on 461 children from a North American multicenter registry. Pediatrics. 2008;122(6):e1128–35.

Perkins JD. Incidence of portal vein complications following liver transplantation. Liver Transpl. 2008;14(12):1813–5.

Perkins JD. Balloon dilation only versus balloon dilation plus stenting for posttransplantation biliary strictures. Liver Transpl. 2009;15(1):106–10.

Pfitzmann R, Nüssler NC, Hippler-Benscheidt M, Neuhaus R, Neuhaus P. Long-term results after liver transplantation. Transpl Int. 2008;21(3):234–46.

Samada Suarez M, Hernández Perera JC, Ramos Robaina L, Barroso Márquez L, González Rapado L, Valdés MC, Rivero HH, Abdo Cuza A, Valdés AR, Pérez Bernal J, Bernardos A. Factors that predict survival in patients with cirrhosis considered for liver transplantation. Transplant Proc. 2008;40(9):2965–7.

Saner FH, Sotiropoulos GC, Radtke A, Fouzas I, Molmenti EP, Nadalin S, Paul A. Intensive care unit management of liver transplant patients: a formidable challenge for the intensivist. Transplant Proc. 2008;40(9):3206–8.

Saner FH, Nadalin S, Radtke A, Sotiropoulos GC, Kaiser GM, Paul A. Liver transplantation and neurological side effects. Metab Brain Dis. 2009;24(1):183–7.

Sotiropoulos GC, Drühe N, Sgourakis G, Molmenti EP, Beckebaum S, Baba HA, Antoch G, Hilgard P, Radtke A, Saner FH, Nadalin S, Paul A, Malagó M, Broelsch CE, Lang H. Liver transplantation, liver resection, and transarterial chemoembolization for hepatocellular carcinoma in cirrhosis: which is the best oncological approach? Dig Dis Sci. 2009;54(10): 2264–73.

Suh KS, Yi NJ, Kim J, Shin WY, Lee HW, Han HS, Lee KU. Laparoscopic hepatectomy for a modified right graft in adult-to-adult living donor liver transplantation. Transplant Proc. 2008;40(10):3529–31.

Townsend DR, Bagshaw SM, Jacka MJ, Bigam D, Cave D, Gibney RT. Intraoperative renal support during liver transplantation. Liver Transpl. 2009;15(1):73–8.

Zhang Y, Wen T, Yan L, Chen Z, Li B, Zeng Y, Zhao J, Wang W, Yang J, Xu M, Ma Y. Clinical significance of detailed preoperative evaluation on donors in right lobe living donor liver transplantation. Hepatogastroenterology. 2008;55(86–87):1725–8.

Index

Printed in the United States
By Bookmasters